INTEGRATIVE MEDICINE

The Professional Guide To Positive Transformation Through Hypnotherapy

Written by:

Edward J Longo

MISSION STATEMENT

Inspire the Injured Spirit and You Can dissipate Any Disorder, Even Disease.

. . . Edward J Longo

Publisher: EbookSites.org

503 East 78th Street

New York, NY 10075

212-737-8538

ebooks@ebooksites.org

Copyright 2013 - Edward J Longo

ISBN 9780971362369

INTEGRATIVE MEDICINE

The Professional Guide To Positive Transformation Through Hypnotherapy.

A BRIEF TESTIMONY

"Within his recent book on hypnotherapy certified hypnotherapist Edward J Longo offers to both novice and professional readers a panoramic 220-page overview of the great value of hypnotherapy in dealing with common life problems such as weight loss, depression, panic disorder and emotional stress. This highly readable book moves from the general nature of hypnosis – the subconscious, the autonomic nervous system, trances, DSM-4, etc. – to specific techniques for hypnotherapy scripts, inductions, affirmations, and even how one can become qualified as a certified hypnotherapist."

Above comment by Harold Takooshian, PhD, of Fordham University
President (2007), Society for General Psychology,
Division One of the American Psychological Association

INTEGRATIVE THINKING

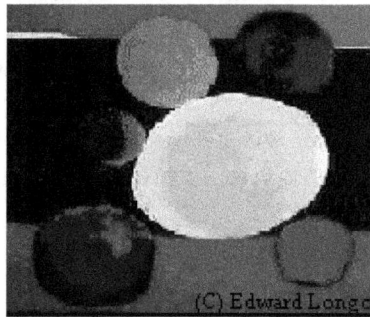

Painting (C) Edward J Longo

INTEGRATIVE MEDICINE

The Professional Guide To Positive Transformation Through Hypnotherapy.

This book is intended to aid professionals such as physicians, lawyers, chiropractors, nurses, social workers, Ph D's, psychotherapists, and other practitioners of varied practices. It is especially valuable for anyone interested in becoming certified as hypnotherapists. Use of this book, other than for the purpose of Integrative Medicine, or The Trance Zone Hypnotherapy is not approved by the author.

Definitions of Integrative Medicine:

http://www.webmd.com/a-to-z-guides/features/alternative-medicine-integrative-medicine

http://www.drweil.com/drw/u/ART02054/Andrew-Weil-Integrative-Medicine.html

http://www.drcmcooke.com/index.php?page=why-integrative-medicine

AUTHOR'S WEBSITES:
http://www.affinityzone.com
http://www.thetrancezone.com
http://www.hypnotherapytoliveby.com
http://integrative-medicine.affinityzone.com

INTEGRATIVE MEDICINE

The Professional Guide To Positive Transformation Through Hypnotherapy.

CONTENTS

The principle of penetrating the subconscious mind is as simple as offering a positive suggestion, a new thought, or a different truth. This locality is where the memory functions at its very best. The subconscious mind is programmed like an endless tape, implanted within the complex synapses and cells of the brain. Actually, one <u>becomes</u> what the subconscious mind thinks. Then, our thoughts and beliefs transform us into our character which aids in complimenting our physiological makeup.

While participating within workings of this <u>*Integrative Medicine*</u> book the subjects, clients, or patients will gain the advantage of gaining unlimited health benefits. This is because you, as hypnotherapist, will introduce them to supernatural powers while demonstrating hypnotic trances in conjunction with the many inductions described within the examples, techniques and illustrations. In refusing to succumb to subversive habits, such as smoking, alcoholism, drug addiction, overeating, and the like, you place the patients' futures on a straight path, healthy and dynamic, toward achieving their ultimate goals.

PART ONE

This chapter explains the history of hypnosis, the basis of hypnotherapy, and a deeper understanding of the subconscious power. Acting as hypnotherapist, WORDS will paint images on the client's mind. The images and demonstrations will aid each practitioner in being able to provide empowerment in an ideal, creative way. In this chapter there will be valuable information about hypnosis, and self-hypnosis. In addition, you will be provided with an uncanny understanding of hypnosis as it relates to the practice of hypnotherapy. This chapter also reveals information about the hypnotic trance state. The objective of the hypnotherapist is to give helpful guidance along with positive images and have them take root in the subconscious mind.

In this chapter participant will also learn, in elaborate detail, all the requirements necessary for inducing hypnosis using *The Trance Zone Hypnotherapy*. Once introduced to the meditative trance you will be amazed how quickly you allow yourself to drift deeper into this warm and beautiful level of your mind. Really, that is all hypnosis is – a purely hypnotic, meditative state of mind. The hypnotic trance state is an altered state of consciousness whereby, as if by some mystical power, the whole psyche shifts into an exaggerated state of positive exuberance. It is similar to that of "the zone" that athletes talk about when an inner force takes over and places the participant into a state where every movement seems effortless.

CONTENTS (continued)

PART TWO

By implementing the information provided within *The Trance Zone Hypnotherapy* you will become able to learn much about the function of hypnosis, self-hypnosis, and even how the process of hypnotherapy is implemented. You will learn how to put subjects into a trance, as well as learn about various mental health issues used to treat patients. Also explained herein is the psychology of hypnotherapy, the states of mind, and the descriptions of the Psychological Tools.

This chapter provides explanations of the hypnotherapist's induction procedures necessary for incorporating the art of hypnotherapy via the hypnotic trance. In addition to instructions on how to *"Go Into" The Trance Zone* examples of trance script inductions are also described and demonstrated in detail. Entering into the trance state is quite a simple process because, after all, hypnosis is merely a state on focused relaxation. It is through this relaxed state that positive results can nearly always be ascertained. Because the conscious mind becomes by-passed, or disarmed, the subconscious readily accepts everything it receives as the TRUTH.

PART THREE

This chapter describes how the mind can alter the brain, and includes insight on altering the belief system. As far as setting the captive free conditioning can go both ways - it can either hold us captive, or it can release us from our bondage. One way to become released from bondage is to practice repetition so positive the mind will come to believe the message as being true. On making positive changes and gaining Psychological Adjustment: positive repetitions, faithfully practiced, will eventually come to be accepted by the mind and become manifest into reality. Because its effect is organic, hypnotherapy is truly a marvel of mind over mind. Used properly, it can be used as a tool to investigate past lives, probe into the problems of the psyche, and even traverse and envision what the future may have in store. By unleashing subconscious powers patients will become enabled with the mind's most effective tool: the hypnotic trance.

The practice of hypnosis for the purpose of enhancing hypnotherapy is not a mere mental procedure. Even to this day, its majestic powers have become a supernatural phenomenon that continues to behoove even the most learned of persons. Being hypnotized to overcome issues is definitely the wave of the future, where more and more people are striving to grow intellectually and psychologically, as well as spiritually. Finally, health, wealth, and the pursuit of happiness can be achieved by all who dare to become involved in one of the most revolutionary forms of treatment of the 21st century. Actual trance scripts performed on patients over a period of fifteen years have been developed for specific patients with the focus on particular issues.

PART FOUR

This chapter provides numerous examples and goes into intricate detail explaining the Induction Techniques used to *"Go Into"* _The Trance Zone_. Here, the hypnotherapist will also learn about Writing Custom Scripts, such as Behavior Modification, the Spinning Crystal Technique, Overcoming Insomnia including , Fulfilling The Subject's Needs For A Trim Waist. Many induction methods, such as how to place the patient into a trance using the "liquid tranquilizer" are also revealed within the context of these powerful hypnotic trance scripts.

As an indication of such incredible positive healng the author presents his mission statement, a statement so effective that he has based his entire treatment on this remarkable concept: *Inspire The Injured Spirit And You Can Dissipate Any Disorder, even Disease.* This chapter continues go into detail explaining behavior modification, and also demonstrates how the hypnotherapist successfully empowers the patient simply through the use of suggestions, and mind-altering affirmations. Illustrations such as The Blue Aura of Dharma, and inductions such as Hypnotic Induction for Empowerment, and Quitting Bad Habits become helpful aids in treating a wide spectrum of disorders.   The 9 Common Myths and Misconceptions will also be introduced.

PART FIVE

Through the introduction of the Surgeon General's mental health report, neuroscience and examples from the DSM-IV manual, the hypnotherapist will finally be able to investigate areas that are likely to instill inspiration, and even provide valuable motivation.   The written material contained herein is not intended to profess being an authority on the entire workings of the mind, or the brain for that matter; (an irresistible pun.) The information provided is solely to invite the hypnotherapist, practitioner, or interested professionals to become subjected to the many ways of gaining access to supreme knowledge, thereby becoming more helpful to mankind.

Through the introduction of the marvelous workings of the Neurological Brain and the Autonomic Nervous System hypnotherapists will be able increase their knowledge base. This complex system consists of sensory neurons and motor neurons that run between the central nervous system (especially the hypothalamus and medulla oblongata) and various internal organs such as: the heart, lungs, viscera glands (both exocrine and endocrine). It is responsible for monitoring conditions in the internal environment and bringing about appropriate changes within them. The contraction of both smooth muscle and cardiac muscle is controlled by motor neurons of the autonomic system. Through the introduction of the marvelous workings of the nervous system and vital information about the workings of the heart, the hypnotherapist will now be able to add more expertise by investigating the important links to psychological and physiological makeup.

CONTENTS (continued)

PART SIX

Chapter 11 - Manifestations of The Highest Kind-
Through learning the secrets of transformation you will finally come to understand hidden meanings. Here, through the use of Trance Manifestations, the hypnotherapist will introduce subjects to luck, while patients are shown how to acquire Manifestations of The Highest Kind. The manifestations listed within, are the forms in which some power, such as a divine being, through thought, or an idea, is revealed. The materialized form of a spirit, or the discovery of the third eye, or to a renewed understanding; everything defined above, plus that which manifests, exhibits, or displays. This is renewed Revelation, as in The Manifestation of God's Power in Creation. Through learning the secrets of attracting luck you will come to understand other hidden meanings.

Chapter 12 - Inducing Majestic Trance Spells
By a special positioning the hands and forming "The Hypnotic Eye," the subject, client, or hypnotherapist, will be able to induce the highly effective, hypnotic, Majestic Trance Spells. Due to the fact that it is not immediately recognizable, deprivation is the primary cause of self-abuse, insomnia, addiction and the consequences of rejection. It is also responsible for inferiority complexes, phobias and obsessive compulsion disorders (OCD,) as well as an entire spectrum of other maladies. Because most victims of deprivation become so caught up in their problems, they become unaware of these influences - they have become blinded, thus creating an inability. In affect, they become powerless and succumb to the dominant forces sabotaging their subconscious. The old saying, "You can't see the forest through the trees" has some truth in it. If you wish to see the big picture, you need to seriously contemplate the layout of the forest.

PART SEVEN

Chapter 13 - Physiotherapy Technique™
Those committing to exercise will find this as the elixir to the mind and spirit, as well as the physical body. In doing so, subjects will be surprised to find it strengthens the will, activates the organs and inspires the spirit. Learn how to gain a healthy body and a sound mind. Through a never-ending responsibility to ourselves, we must see to it that our bodies get the proper exercise and nourishment, enough so that it becomes a sustaining fuel - a progressive blood / cell regeneration process. This physical conditioning is our only way of retarding the inevitable pull towards death. In fact, in the animal kingdom, the expression "the survival of the fittest" is truly representative of their way of life. In their world, the weak are always the first to succumb. It is the same in our world – death holds a ringside seat and continues to beckon the underdog called "self-neglect," while life, "the fittest" opponent, spars to defend the title of longevity.

Chapter 14 - The Trance Zone Hypnotherapy Course
Being the modality whose time has come, it is already taking a positive affect in society as The Alternative Therapy of The Future. In participating in this new wave of positive transformation, physical and emotional healing will be standard for strengthening the will, activating the organs and most importantly, inspiring the spirit. After reviewing the chapters within why not seriously consider becoming a certified hypnotherapist. **Think Career!**

CONTENTS (continued)

APPENDIX A

After 20 years working as a certified hypnotherapist and treating patients for a wide variety or disorders based on "*The Trance Zone Hypnosis Manual*," I realized I had developed enough material for even a 2nd non-fiction book. This became: *The Trance Zone Hypnotherapy Course - Hypnotherapy Certification.*

Phase One Includes the history of hypnosis, self-hypnosis and conditioning, understanding the subconscious mind, how to reach and arouse the Genie within, the Secret 7 Golden Rules, Insight of Mental Energy, structuring successful suggestions, and the ethics of practice. Phase One also includes numerous induction techniques, testing for depth of hypnotic trance, stress tests, and how to treat smoking addiction, obesity, lack of confidence, self-esteem, nail biting, stuttering, Tourette's Syndrome, and so much more.

Phase Two Consists of the learned experiences of becoming a certified hypnotist as described above, including the understanding and application of the deep hypnotic states of mind. Here, you will become enabled to address anxiety, health and well being, deepening trance techniques, advanced treatment for specific emotional problems and illnesses, developing and delivering hypnotic scripts, stress management, Spiritual Steam, Electromagnetism, responsibilities of the professional hypnotherapist, (including operating your practice, fees, referrals, etc.,) implanting positive suggestions, including guided imagery enabling you to become a master practitioner. Yes, even becoming empowered physically as well as spiritually, in order to provide health solutions all throughout your career. And finally: registration with the American Board of Hypnotherapy using The Trance Zone Hypnotherapy Certificate as a viable, highly credible credential.

APPENDIX B

This appendix provides information on how to become certified in nearly every state in America. Since it has been announced that college tuition may be well over $60,000.00 per year to become a student of the New York University, why not seriously consider a career as a board certified hypnotherapist? Why spend four to eight years getting an education when, upon the completion of this course, you could easily begin earning $75 to $150 per hour and up within the first year. Why not give consideration of having a legal, hypnotherapy certificate in your name.

FORWARD

FORWARD:

Integrative Medicine Defined

Integrative medicine is the use of complementary, alternative, holistic, and "natural," preventive practices. Implementing integrative health includes a varied array of modalities, such as acupressure, yoga, homeotherapy, meditation, hypnotherapy, and cognitive therapy that are not considered part of "conventional" medicine.

Man finds himself isolated in the cosmos, because he is no longer involved in nature and has lost his emotional 'unconscious identity' with natural phenomena. These have lost their symbolic implications.

His contact with nature has gone, and with it has gone the profound emotional energy that his symbolic connection supplied.

. . . Carl Jung

FORWARD

EVERYTHING WE ARE
COMES FROM THE SUBCONSCIOUS

So, what can hypnotherapy do for you? Not only can hypnosis be used to improve your physical and mental functioning, but it can also be used as a tool to achieve a great level of success and self-esteem for your clients. Although being under hypnosis is not in any way harmful, it is understandable that someone may be slightly apprehensive their first time. After one or two visits with an experienced hypnotherapist, persons will come to realize that hypnosis is a very helpful tool and a wondrous, healthy way to arm themselves for the 21st century.

The principle of penetrating the subconscious mind is as simple as offering a positive suggestion, a new thought, or a different truth. This is where the memory functions at its very best. The subconscious mind is programmed like an endless tape, implanted within the complex synapses and atomic cells of the brain. Actually, you become what your subconscious mind thinks. Then, our thoughts and beliefs transform us into our character and give us our psychological makeup.

You may think you can always consciously control your emotions, but after experiencing a crisis you may have wondered why you behaved so erratically, even sporadically. Actually, your subconscious mind is in control of every function necessary to keep you alive and well; functions that the conscious mind is not aware of performing. Try maintaining your heart rate, your blood count, your cell structure, and how many times you blink every minute of the day – all at the same time. (A little known fact is that the eyes even move and blink during sleep.)

How about taking complete control of your memory? Properly accessed, it is possible to go into that subconscious tape and play back every word; every picture; every incident you've ever experienced – even from the very day you were born. In fact, the trauma of birth has had, in some ways, a lasting effect on each and every person. Going beyond that, since the subconscious is Ancestral in development, it actually becomes feasible to access past lives – this is because the subconscious is also supernatural in spirit.

The good news is that, even after death, the spirit continues to live on – for the spirit is eternal. According to Einstein, energy never dies. Why would anyone in their right mind want to argue with that?

THE COLLECTIVE UNCONSCIOUS Verses
THE COLLECTIVE SUBCONSCIOUS

The Collective Unconscious:

Carl Jung's term, *"the collective unconscious"* essentially represents archetype individuals, universally, in their present state of mind – suggesting that the human psyche is connected universally, but not necessarily, ancestrally.

The Collective Subconscious, or Super-conscious:

According to The Trance Zone Hypnotherapy, "the collective subconscious" is actually representative of persons universally, as well as ancestrally, in a highly spiritual state of mind – meaning that all living persons have the potential to connect super-consciously. Therefore, the super-conscious state is representative, not only of persons as they exist in their present, carnal state, but as they have progressed from their ancestral, reincarnate state, as well.

In fact, this super-conscious state has the metabolic, electromagnetic capacity of continuing exceedingly into the future as *"The source"* of spiritual energy. Through evolution and genetics, certain characteristics of temperament and emotions run through bloodlines quite similar to that of horses, and other animals. *(For more on this, see The Emotional Brain, by Joseph Le Doux.)*

The above information can also be explained and clarified within the works of Gautama Buddha, the pages of The Tibetan Book of the Dead, the Koran, and within Cayce's readings on Atlantis.

The Seven Spiritual Centers:

In Yoga terminology, the seven chakra centers of the snakelike Kundalini are coiled, or lined up within the body from the top of the head to the base of the spine: Crown Chakra; Third Eye Chakra; Throat Chakra; Heart Chakra; Solar Plexus Chakra; Sacral Chakra; and the base Root Chakra.

The Endocrine Glands:

The Endocrine Glands pertaining to our health and wellbeing are as follows: the pituitary, pineal, thyroid, thymus, adrenals, Leydig cells, and the testes or ovaries.

The Triune Brain:

Paul MacLean, the former director of the Laboratory of the Brain and Behavior at the United States National Institute of Mental Health, developed a model of the brain based on its evolutionary development. This was referred to as the "triune brain theory" because he suggested that the human brain was actually three-brains-in-one. Each of the layers, or "brains," was established successively in response to evolutionary need. The three layers are the reptilian system, or *R-complex*, the *limbic system*, and the *neocortex*. Each layer is geared toward separate functions of the brain, but all three layers interact substantially. Below are partial descriptions:

The Reptilian Complex

The R-complex consists of the brain stem and the cerebellum. Its purpose is closely related to actual physical survival and maintenance of the body. The cerebellum orchestrates movement.

The Limbic System

The limbic system, the second brain to evolve, houses the primary centers of emotion. It includes the amygdala, which is important in the association of events with emotion, and the hippocampus, which is active in converting information into memory and memory recall. Some neuroscientists believe that the hippocampus helps select which memories are stored, perhaps by attaching an "emotion marker" to some events so that they are likely to be recalled. The amygdala comes into play in situations that arouse feelings such as fear, pity, anger, or outrage.

The Neocortex

Also called the cerebral cortex, constitutes five-sixths of the human brain. It is the outer portion of our brain, and is approximately the size of a crumpled newspaper page. The neocortex makes language, including speech and writing possible. It renders logical and formal operational thinking possible and allows us to see ahead and plan for the future.

Resource: *Caine, Renate Nummela and Geoffrey Caine. Making Connections: Teaching and the Human Brain. Nashville, TN: Incentive Publications, 1990*

INTRODUCTION

INTRODUCTION:

By utilizing the principles of The Trance Zone Hypnotherapy you will not only gain the opportunity to improve the mind of others; you will be enabled with such power you will become alive, more so than you have ever dreamed. The secret to tapping the depths of the mind is to go into the subconscious, where the true source of power rules.

Here, you become enabled to unleash the power of the subconscious mind in order change negative habits of thought and action into what you desire them to be – especially in regard to treating patients. This is where, and how, you can begin reprogramming the mind in order to utilize the brain's unfathomable resources. This highly creative approach to hypnotherapy provides an intellectual powerhouse, regarding mastery of the mind. More importantly, hypnotherapy initiates the total performance of the capabilities of the subconscious within the triune brain, especially upon initiating "The Hypnotic Eye."

Edward J Longo - Board Certified Hypnotherapist

INTRODUCTION

THE TRANCE ZONE HYPNOTHERAPY
THE NUMEROUS BENEFITS

The Trance Zone Hypnotherapy became developed out of a need to put into practice my experiences with human behavior under complex situations, which included the study of personalities, and the correlation between varied attitudes, underlying thoughts and innate intentions, whether superficial or genuine. Encompassing more than 25 years, I have been researching the psychological relevance between the conscious and the subconscious mind. Throughout these extensive life experiences, which included the study of acting; being a chauffeur for the rich and famous; and having the opportune observation of a wide variety of personalities, I finally became qualified and then certified as a board certified hypnotherapist.

Through my understanding of the miracles Jesus performed through His remarkable spirit, it is of my opinion that He possessed, not only the powers of a healer and psychologist, but of a hypnotherapist as well. What He did, primarily, was to heal and cast out demons, so no matter where Jesus went He performed a miracle. This was His supernatural gift from God.

The fact that the term "Christ Consciousness" has evolved makes this even more convincing. Obviously, Jesus Christ possessed the highest knowledge of the subconscious mind, as well as possessing supernatural powers of the highest kind. Just what kind of state of mind did Jesus create? Well, through extensive research of the bible, I have concluded that, in order to induce His healing powers, He had the gift of being able to create the highest spiritual state of mind possible – to which I deem must have been the divine, trance state, or The Absolute Trance. This is why I profess "*The Trance Zone hypnotic state is the closest one can get to God without dying.*"

(continue)

THE NUMEROUS BENEFITS (continued)

Truthfully, I don't profess to have such powers, but through my discovery of this revelation, I became interested in the spiritual world, as well as the need to implement such powers to thwart threats that surround us in this physical realm. And, yes, I do believe in the devil and his workings. This is why I feel so strong about working with the subconscious mind, for I have come to believe that all disease and mental problems are caused by the influence of negative forces – some lesser, some increasingly pronounced by the dark and sinister, evil forces.

Without reservation, I can honestly say that this is why I believe my work to be of a supernatural nature. Not unlike Jesus, in some regard, I always look to my God to intercede, whether I am teaching, working, or performing my hypnotherapy through the use of deep hypnosis, or through incorporating the divine practice of *The Absolute Trance,* herein established as *The Trance Zone.*

Due to all the damaging, negative influences bombarding us from all fronts, hypnotherapists within this alternative health field are becoming more respected, and will inevitably become much more in demand . . . EJL

WHAT YOU ARE CAPABLE OF ACCOMPLISHING AS A HYPNOTHERAPIST:

While participating within the workings of this *Integrative Medicine* book the subjects, clients, or patients will gain the advantage of gaining unlimited health benefits. This is because you, as hypnotherapist, will introduce them to supernatural powers while demonstrating hypnotic trances in conjunction with the many inductions described within the examples, techniques and illustrations. In refusing to succumb to subversive habits, such as smoking, alcoholism, drug addiction, overeating, and the like, you place the patients' futures on a straight path, healthy and dynamic, toward achieving their ultimate goals.

The psychosomatic energy incurred by alleviating the many degenerative habits will boost their confidence and energy levels to such a degree it will induce transformation and in turn, manifest their ideals, wishes, desires, and innermost dreams. Conversely, to succumb to any form of life-sapping habit is tantamount to being unable to resist a dark glass of anti-matter presented by death's own hand. Degenerative habits are the devil's invented diversions to personal gain, needs, self-esteem, heart's desires, and all forms of positive energies associated with the progression of life-giving forces. The key is to seek and develop constraint – better yet, cessation of all negative vices, and devices.

THE TRANCE ZONE DEFINED

EXACTLY WHAT IS THE TRANCE ZONE?

In addition to valuable information, possibly leading to hypnotherapy certification, Edward J Longo, an ABH certified hypnotherapist, provides the principles of self-hypnosis as well as mock hypnosis sessions for the purpose of illustrating private treatments. Each candidate will learn basic, practitioner services, which include physical, spiritual and mental indoctrination. Expert techniques will be introduced as a possibility of reducing anxiety disorders, panic attacks, depression, mental abuse, bipolar, mania, personality disorders, physical and mental dysfunction, OCD, phobias, memory loss, stress, and other health issues.

Also, many techniques will be introduced that are intended to enable the candidate to induce private sessions for the purpose of treating patients. Due to the extensive background of this master hypnotherapist much insight will, invariably, be illustrated and demonstrated throughout this book. Fortunately, there is a psychotherapist's book that provides vital information on the principles of alleviating, or warding off, disease and mental disorders. This book is a practical guide to positive transformation, which is appropriately named:

Integrative Medicine,
The Professional Guide To Positive Transformation Through Hypnotherapy.

The Trance Zone, otherwise described as *"The Absolute Trance"* is that deepened, subconscious state of mind where the adrenaline, metabolism, visual perception and intuition becomes increased, inducing the elated feeling of being in the groove. As this state of arousal kicks in it then becomes referred to as being in *"the zone,"* as many athletes have reported. This is the point whereby hypnosis then becomes organic in nature, and therefore everything seems to be functioning as if nothing could go wrong. Indeed, "going into" the trance state gives one the feeling that everything is sure to turn out just right. Going even beyond *"the zone,"* and then arriving into that highly spiritual source is that place where the participant knows everything will turn out perfect. This is that spiritual place deep within where the participant experiences the supernatural connection to *"the source."* That source has been established as *"The Trance Zone."*

(continue)

EXACTLY WHAT IS THE TRANCE ZONE? (continued)

According to Aquarian philosophy Akashia is the first stage of spiritual crystallization. This philosophy recognizes the fact that all Primary, or primordial substance, is spiritual and moving at a lower rate of vibration, becoming a profound source of energy. This Akashic, or Primary substance, is of exquisite fineness and is so sensitive that the slightest vibrations of an ether anywhere in the universe register an indelible impression upon it.

This primal substance is not relegated to any particular part of the universe, but is everywhere present. It is, in fact, the Spirit of Supreme Intelligence, The Super-conscious, or the Universal Mind, of which metaphysicians speak. When the mind is in exact accord with this omnipotent energy it enters into a subconscious recognition of these Akashic impressions, and may collect and translate them into any language on earth with which the individual is familiar.

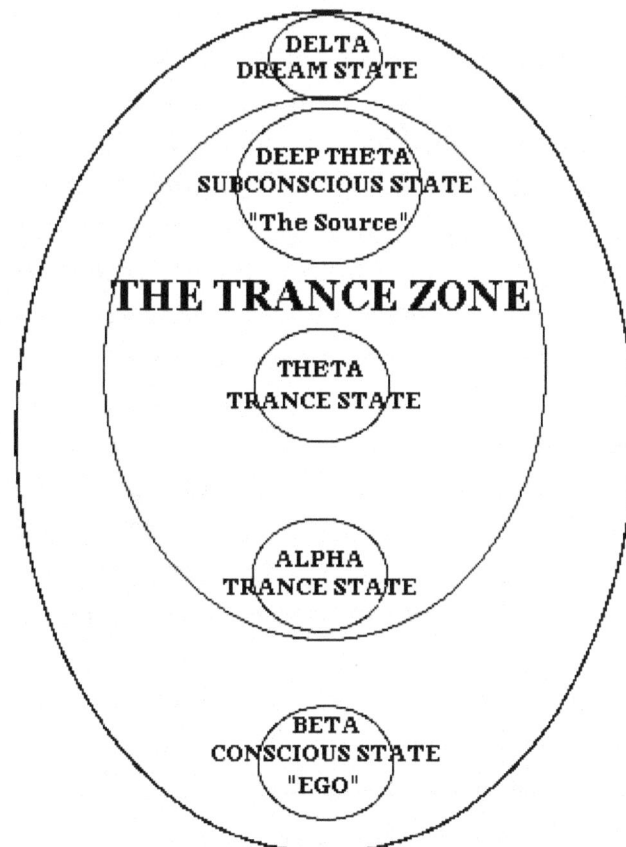

DELTA
DREAM STATE

DEEP THETA
SUBCONSCIOUS STATE
"The Source"

THE TRANCE ZONE

THETA
TRANCE STATE

ALPHA
TRANCE STATE

BETA
CONSCIOUS STATE
"EGO"

THE MIND BRAIN WAVES

The most incomprehensible aspect of the subconscious, "The Source" of The Supernatural Power, is that it IS comprehensible.   (continue)

EXACTLY WHAT IS THE TRANCE ZONE? (continued)

The Trance Zone Hypnotherapy:

By utilizing the principles of *The Trance Zone Hypnotherapy* you will not only gain the opportunity to improve the mind of others; you will be enabled with such power you will become alive, more so than you have ever dreamed. The secret to tapping the depths of the mind is to go into the subconscious, where the true source of power rules. Here, you become enabled to unleash the power of the subconscious mind in order change negative habits of thought and action into what you desire them to be – especially in regard to treating patients. This is where, and how, you can begin reprogramming the mind in order to utilize the brain's unfathomable resources. This highly creative approach to hypnotherapy provides an intellectual powerhouse, regarding mastery of the mind.

The Trance Zone Hypnotherapy provides that kind of dynamics. The theory behind this technique is one intended to stimulate that part of the psyche, which brings the participant, or subject, to that very pinnacle. It is designed to enlist that pinnacle where, seemingly, nothing is impossible, nothing can go wrong, or interfere with achieving only the best results. The most important thing about hypnosis is that the nervous system cannot tell the difference between real and imagined experiences. By gaining access to the subconscious you can induce a trance and go anywhere, achieve anything, or be anyone you wish to become.

In utilizing *The Trance Zone Hypnotherapy* you have the benefit of altering minds to the degree persons don't have to struggle with quitting smoking, addiction, or any other dysfunction. When you succeed at developing self-esteem and see subjects transformed as a more perfect and complete human being, all those bad, negative gremlins simply fade away. In these hypnotic states of healing, everything becomes simple – yet nothing is ever impossible.

Upon bypassing the conscious state, you will eventually access the unlimited attributes of the altered, subconscious state. The process of accessing the subconscious mind can be that simple when using the principles demonstrated within *The Trance Zone Hypnotherapy.*

(continue)

EXACTLY WHAT IS THE TRANCE ZONE? (continued)

Psychological Tools - Eight Hypnotic Aids:

Listed below, are descriptions of the two major psychological tools suggested in order to induce hypnosis in *The Trance Zone.*

All eight tools are presented later in detail within Chapter 3 in the following order: *The hypnotic eye; eyes up to the eyebrows; deep yawn; inhale through the nose;* and *Hypnotic WORDS*. Alternative tools include *subliminal sounds; movement; and The Insight of Mental Imagery.*

The Hypnotic Eye

The posturing of the fingers has been commonly perceived as a sign indicating that everything is okay. Holding the hand in the air, indicating with the encircled thumb and forefinger has been widely used to represent many kinds of expressions, including perfection, to stress a point, or to demonstrate confidence. It has also been used to demonstrate security, or to express positive feelings. Regarding its role in *The Trance Zone*, *"the hypnotic eye,"* or The Third Eye, is used to trigger the connection to The Source, called *"The Supernatural Power."*

During hypnotherapy sessions the subject, or patient, is advised that, when forming *"the hypnotic eye"* they become connected to *"the eye to the subconscious, which is the direct link to The Supernatural Power."*

(See Chapter 3, **Illustration 3-2** under Psychological Tools.)

The Third Eye

The finest vibrations which we have yet considered are within the realm of the electrical and magnetic phenomena. There are forces which man also contains within himself, and which can be utilized through the mind. We must not inquire what organs man has with which to register these particular vibrations, embracing the radiations and emanations which come under the general term "psychic." There are two small glands in the head which give doctors much cause for speculation. I refer to the Pituitary Body and the Pineal Gland.

The former is a tiny, double bean-shaped body situated behind the root of the nose. It is posed so that it is very sensitive to vibrations. We know that it is in some way connected with the nurture, body-building and the nervous system. If it is removed all organic function ceases.

<u>The Third Eye</u> (continued)

If overdeveloped it produces giantism, while if underdeveloped dwarfism is the result. The Pituitary Body has been called the seat on the mind. Its frontal lobe is concerned with emotional thought, of the type which produces poetry and music; while the anterior lobe is connected with more concrete intellectual concepts.

The Pineal Gland is a tiny cone-shaped body in the middle of the head, behind and just above the Pituitary. It contains pigment similar to that found in the eyes, and is connected by two nerve cords with the optic thalmi; it is said to control the action of light upon the body, and for the reasons scientists have suggested that it is the remnant of a third physical eye. Men of learning, such as Descartes, have pronounced to be the point in the human being where the soul and body meet, the soul of intuition.

It is said that when, for specific reasons, the Pituitary Body and the Pineal Gland have become fully developed and stimulated, their vibrations fuse and stir into life the mysterious "Third Eye" of man, the eye to the soul. Apparently this activity provides the mind with a perfect instrument with which to work, a transmitter by means of which vibrations of very differing types can be translated, interpreted and rearranged.

Resource: *The Finding of the Third Eye* by Vera Stanley Adler.
Note: This fine book may be included as part of the *Trance Zone Hypnotherapy Course* with permission as granted by Weiser Books.

Also Note: *The Trance Zone* hypnosis concept was conceptualized prior to any knowledge of the existence of *The Finding of the Third Eye*. The remarkable thing about this was when I discovered how closely these two unique concepts wound up so interrelated. The only way I can explain this phenomenon is that it is just another illustration of how closely we are connected as a whole within the collective subconscious state. To my mind, this could also explain how profoundly linked we are to our ancestral counterparts in present, or past lives, supernaturally

. . . Edward J Longo

PART ONE

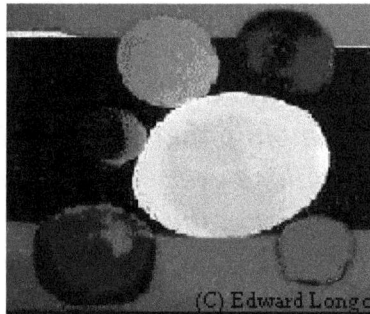

CHAPTER ONE
1

HYPNOSIS &
HYPNOTHERAPY

---

1 HYPNOSIS AS THE BASIS OF
HYPNOTHERAPY:

Hypnosis: The technique of gaining access to a person's subconscious state of mind – in this case, using The Trance Zone and, "the hypnotic eye" technique. Whatever you do in life, there's always one weapon that's there to back you up. One weapon so powerful, life changing, and impact filled that it can determine the difference between success and failure every single time you use it.
In business, this weapon either gets you the sale or it doesn't.
The power it supplies is directly dependant on the ammunition that YOU provide. That weapon lies within you as the power of hypnotherapy." . . . EJL

Hypnotherapist – Through the Hypnotherapist, words will paint images on the subconscious mind. These images will aid in mastering control over lives in creative and ideal ways. During the process of positive suggestions and Guided Imagery subjects will not become under anyone's control; rather, through unleashing the innate unconscious powers they will become enabled with the Hypnotherapist's most powerful tool – namely:

*Hypnotherapy: In the state of hypnosis, the subconscious mind becomes fully accessible, processing two hundred million sensory messages every second. Conversely, in the conscious state, the mind is less than ten percent operational, processing only a handful of instructions at any given time. **Definition**: Hypnotherapist (hypno-therapist,) a practitioner who uses hypnosis to treat persons for disorders, or mental health issues; a therapist who uses hypnosis to induce therapeutic healing. This is the primary function of the Hypnotherapist.*

CHAPTER ONE
1

HYPNOSIS &
HYPNOTHERAPY

HYPNOSIS
The Basis For Initiating Hypnotherapy

What Exactly IS Hypnosis?

Hypnosis has a reputation of being harmful because of bad press, hearsay and a whole range of misunderstandings. The hypnotist is often seen as a dark, maniacal character that inflicts his will upon victims through hypnotic powers. Amateur stage hypnotists, horror movies, and fear of the unknown have caused much of the misinformation. In actuality, many people should be more concerned about what their negative, conscious state dictates, rather than fearing what hypnotherapy can do to transform them in such a positive way.

The fact of the matter is that hypnotherapy truly represents a different story. Hypnotherapy, through the professional use of hypnosis, is a natural, relaxed state of mind and body similar to that of a daydream. This is the state of mind that enables one, if so desired, to use the imagination to help effect positive changes. Although the swinging pocket watch had been associated with hypnosis, it is still associated with controlling a person's behavior – just as the myth about being taken over and controlled against one's will is equally unfounded. In essence, it is always the subject, client, or patient, who is in control – not the hypnotherapist. The hypnotherapist simply induces hypnosis with positive verbal suggestions, reinforcing them with colorful, guided imagery.

(continue)

<u>HYPNOSIS</u> (continued)

A Brief History About Hypnosis:

Hypnosis sometimes occurs automatically, whether you are aware of it or not. This is the inherent state of mind where perception, ideas, and daydreams occur regularly. For example: You are cruising along in you car, lost in your worldly thoughts, when you suddenly arrive at your destination. You haven't the faintest idea of how you got there. The truth is that, since you've driven along this path so many times before, your subconscious mind had memorized the entire route. In effect, you were placed in the hypnotic state. How did you get into the hypnotic state? Were you asleep? Of course not! The fact of the matter is that you were a lot more alert than you realized – that magnificent trance state of your mind shifted into automatic pilot, since your conscious mind became focused somewhere else. Hypnotherapy, then, becomes the process of disarming.

That's the key: <u>focused</u> attention – that is where the subconscious mind comes into play. When the conscious mind becomes completely engrossed in something, the subconscious mind kicks in automatically and takes over. Why does this happen? The trance state becomes activated because the conscious mind can only concentrate on one thing at a time, so when things get complicated the subconscious has to intercede. That's what happens when you are under hypnosis. Since your conscious mind becomes easily distracted, your unconscious mind becomes activated by what's being said – you begin to engage the most productive part of cerebellum. The juices begin to flow, creativity becomes predominant, and your mind becomes susceptible to all kinds of images and positive suggestions.

Hypnosis has been a part of every culture since the inception of the intellectual man. Four thousand years before Christ the Sumerians were already practicing it. In India's book of the Law of Manu an ancient Sanskrit refers to hypnotism as "the ecstatic sleep." Ancient Egypt used hypnosis as a therapeutic measure, exhibited on the Ebers Papyrus. In fact, Egyptian priests had their patients fixate on metal disks until so fatigued they went into hypnotic trance.
Oddly enough, in the eleventh century, monks of the Hesichastic Order, cloistered on Mount Athos and inaugurated the principle of self-hypnosis by contemplating their navels.

(continue)

<u>HYPNOSIS</u> (continued)

Hypnotism was refereed to as "Mesmerism" in the 1700's when Franz Anton Mesmer became known as the father of hypnotherapy. He believed that his "animal fluid," described as "Fluidum," could be stored up in magnets and transferred to patients to cure them of illness. He believed his "fluid" was transmitted by "passes" – making hand movements from top to bottom along the body. The Austrian doctor recognized this ancient healing phenomenon and incorporated it into his theory of "Animal Magnetism."

But Mesmer eventually discarded the magnets. He regarded himself as having the magnetic force. Thousands of sick but hopeful people flocked to his treatment center and he had a tremendous rate of success. However, his theory of Animal Fluid finally became discredited and ridiculed.

"Mesmerism" became the forerunner of hypnotic suggestion, although his cures were attributed only to the imagination. Magnets are still used to relieve pain and discomfort, facilitate healing of broken bones, and the health industry is using MRI's (magnetic resonance imaging) to replace x-rays because it is safer and more effective.

Note: As far as the state of hypnosis, people still refer to finding themselves under a spell, or going into a trance, as being "mesmerized."

How Is The Trance Zone Reached?

Certified Hypnotherapist, Edward J Longo, uses his voice to relax the muscles, thereby inducing the hypnotic trance state of hypnosis. Hypnotherapy, which is hypnosis applied to therapy (i.e., hypno-therapy,) is one of the most effective, alternative practices used today, and it is rapidly growing in acceptance. What can be more beneficial than a caring professional skillfully guiding, and suggesting ways to grow physiologically, mentally, emotionally, and even spiritually, as well?

The experience of the trance is that, because of feeling so mentally and physically unwound, subjects express that it was like being on a mini-vacation. In this state, patients will find it easier to access past events, or memories. The most common evidence of being in the hypnotic state is time distortion, where much more time has elapsed than expected. This is generally due to the relief of the tremendous pressures accumulated over long periods of time.

(continue)

HYPNOSIS (continued)

Although remaining completely aware of their surroundings, persons, experience subconscious changes while in this deepened state of hypnosis, and can converse quite easily even though their eyes are closed. Once this deep state is reached, subjects usually experience a surprising sense of security. And while it is important to maintain a sense of relaxation, it is equally important note that the subject is always made to feel better at end of the session. Hypnotherapy is actually a heightened form of meditation, the only difference being that the hypnotherapist is providing all the right words, and influencing positive images.

Is the Hypnotic Trance Safe?

Hypnosis is absolutely safe because the patient is always in total control. There is no possibility of being manipulated, because the session may be stopped at any time merely by opening one's eyes. The belief that persons may go so deep they will remain in the trance, or possibly lose their minds, is more hearsay. Persons who are placed into hypnosis do not become 'asleep' – in fact they are even more aware of what is taking place than usual. The worse thing that can happen is that the patient may fall asleep, only to awaken automatically a short period later. No one goes into such a deep sleep that they never come out of it. Because of being connected to the powerful subconscious state, the senses function much more efficiently than in the conscious state. Anyone (except the truly mentally subnormal, very young children and inebriates) has the potential to enter the hypnotic state. Persons who have a fear of 'Being put under' or 'Blurting out their secrets' have been misconceived about what hypnosis really is. Reaching the hypnotic state does not mean 'Being put under' – rather, the subject harmlessly 'Goes Into' the trance state.

Hypnosis is not the sleep state, but an altered state of consciousness where our mental images, far deeper than our thoughts, aid in controlling our lives. This is the state of deep relaxation in mind and body commonly known as the trance state. The objective of the hypnotherapist is to give helpful guidance along with positive images and have them take root in the subconscious mind. The end result of the learned experience is that you will become empowered to be master of your own fate.

UNDERSTANDING HYPNOTHERAPY

Hypnotherapy:

Through the Hypnotherapist, words will begin to paint images on the subconscious mind. These images will aid in mastering control over lives in creative and ideal ways. During the process of positive suggestions and <u>Guided Imagery</u> subjects will not become under any control; rather, through unleashing the innate subconscious powers they will become enabled with the hypnotherapist's most powerful tool – hypnotherapy. In the state of hypnosis, the subconscious mind becomes fully accessible, processing two hundred million sensory messages every second. Conversely, in the conscious state, the mind is less than ten percent operational, processing only a handful of instructions at any given time.

During the process of positive suggestions, accompanied with guided imagery, subjects will not become under any control; rather, through unleashing the innate unconscious powers they will become enabled with the hypnotherapist's most powerful tool – hypnotherapy. In the state of hypnosis, the subconscious mind becomes fully accessible, processing two hundred million sensory messages every second. Conversely, in the conscious state, the mind is less than ten percent operational, processing only a handful of instructions at any given time.

What Is The Mystery About Hypnotherapy?

Again, whatever you do in life, there's always one weapon that can always be there to back you up. A weapon so life changing, powerful, and effective that it can make the difference between success and failure. Once you understand, and apply the concept of *The Trance Zone Hypnotherapy* it will work every single time you decide to use it. The key is that you decide. So, what Is This Powerful Secret Weapon?

The answer: WORDS! But WORDS that are suggestive, WORDS that are Positive and Inducted into the Subconscious Mind. Words used otherwise can become exceedingly dangerous – one wrong word to a child can turn happiness into tears. WORDS Are the Life-blood of Communication, as well as Absolute Transformation. Words, whether written or audible, are used to portray thoughts, feelings, emotions, ideas, and ever so much more. They bridge the gap between the conscious and the subconscious, and always provide infinite possibilities.

(continue)

__UNDERSTANDING HYPNOTHERAPY__ (continued)

Yet this secret weapon that is freely available to all is much too often misused, misunderstood, or entirely misinterpreted. The good news is that, instinctively, people love to be engulfed, surrounded, and entertained by words used in stories, speaking, and tales expressed in books. That's why advertising and the media are such booming industries. That's why people read newspapers – it's why people love reading about stories they've experienced themselves. And the more the person can become a confident story teller the more people will become attracted to that voice, that personality, that entertainer, or yes, even that hypnotherapist.

(Note: Please be advised that any attempt to use these hypnotherapy procedures in a harmful, or evil way will only backfire on the person violating the moral principles of hypnosis. Any attempt to harm anyone will be thwarted by the vary person who is attempting to violate these principles.)

Hypnosis began receiving serious study during the 1800's and it was during this period that it received its name. An English ophthalmologist James Braid coined the word, "hypnosis", derived from the Greek word, Hypnos, which means sleep. Braid also showed that hypnotized subjects were very impressionable due to suggestions given verbally. Hypnosis was being used to perform more than 1800 surgical operations painlessly, in London. In India it was commonly used as the sole anesthesia for major operations, such as amputation of limbs.

Autosuggestion became Emile Coue's doctrine during 1857-1926. He claimed that the hypnotist creates an image of the desired effect in the patient's subconscious, and that primarily the patient brings it about. He also claimed that each individual is a powerful hypnotist. "Learn to cure yourself," he would say to his patients. *"You can do it. I have never cured anyone. This power is within you. Call on your mind for help. Make it the servant of your mental and physical well being. It will be present; it will heal you. You will be happy."* He would also direct his patients to repeat the following affirmation twenty times, morning and evening: *"Every day, in every way, I get better and better."* Accordingly, this generated a conditioned reflex, and therefore would become identified with the patient's personality.

(continue)

UNDERSTANDING HYPNOTHERAPY (continued)

In the early 1890's Sigmund Freud, the father of modern psychiatry, used hypnosis in his own practices and even delivered two papers on it. But by the late 1890's he began rejecting hypnosis in favor of his own theories, free association and dream interpretation. So with the rise of psychoanalysis in the first half of this century, hypnosis declined in popularity. But then a reversal occurred. Beginning in the 1950's hypnosis experienced a rebirth. In 1955 the British Medical Association approved the use of hypnotherapy as a valid medical treatment. And in 1958 the American Medical Association (AMA) followed suit. There are now more than 15,000 professionals who use hypnosis in their practices. Recent studies show that 94% of patients benefit from hypnosis, even if the only benefit is relaxation.

During May 1998, three of New York City's most prestigious institutions – Beth Israel Medical Center, Columbia-Presbyterian Memorial Center, and Memorial Sloan-Kettering Cancer Center have announced ambitious plans for programs that promise to feature mind-body medicine. During recent years, there have been many developmental stages of "hooking up" with the Dalai Lama to learn more about Tibetan meditation.

Psychotherapy: Just Another Way to Rewire The Brain

Freud's psychoanalytic theory and the various conditioning theories all assume that anxiety is the result of traumatic learning experiences that foster the establishment of anxiety-producing long-term memories. In this sense psychoanalytic and conditioning theories have drawn similar conclusions about the origins of anxiety.

However, the two kinds of theories lead to different therapeutic approaches. Psychoanalysis seems to help make the patient conscious of the origins of inner conflict, whereas behavior therapy, the name given to therapies inspired by conditioning theories, tries to rid the person of the symptoms of anxiety, often through the various forms of extinction therapy. There is a good deal of debate about the best treatment strategy: psychoanalysis, behavioral therapy, or most recently, cognitive therapy. However, extinction therapies, either alone or in combination with other approaches, are commonly recommended for many anxiety disorders.

Resource: *The Emotional Brain The Mysterious Underpinnings of Emotional Life*
by Joseph LeDoux

UNDERSTANDING HYPNOTHERAPY (continued)

THE ALPHA AND THETA TRANCE STATES

The Trance Zone technique is clearly amidst the new wave toward the practice and understanding of hypnotherapy. Within a short period, you will come to find that the mystery surrounding hypnosis is no mystery at all – that the understanding of hypnosis, after all said and done, has been deluded by shortcomings, shallow-mindedness, and much misconception. The subconscious mind encompasses the entire mind, whether conscious, in the trance state, or completely asleep for the night.

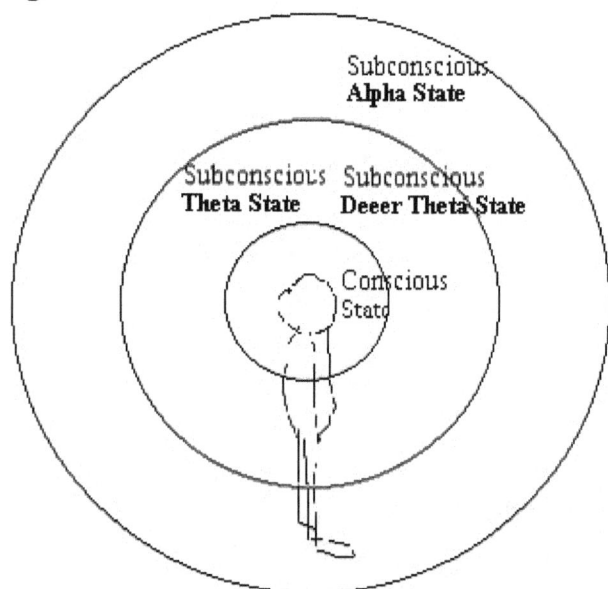

The Three Primary Subconscious Trance States

Although the subconscious mind can never stop processing and operating, terminating only in death, it can shut down as it does when it goes into its deepest sleep mode. When the mind is fully awake, in the conscious state, it is still controlled by the subconscious mind; it is not even able to control how many times the eye blinks every minute. But it is a cinch for the subconscious – it performs billions of tasks without conscious awareness. It does all this automatically – and this is how the conscious mind can be reprogrammed through hypnotherapy.

Regarding the hypnotic trance states there are, primarily, three levels ranging between 4 and 13 Cycles Per Second. They are listed below as follows: the **Subconscious Alpha State**, the **Subconscious Theta State** and the **Subconscious Deeper Theta State.** *(More about this can be found in Chapter Three.)*

UNDERSTANDING HYPNOTHERAPY (continued)

Although most people would disagree, more than 80% of subjects are able to become hypnotized into the lesser **Subconscious Theta State** needed to "go into" the hypnotic trance. Under hypnosis, the hypnotherapist may influence the subject with guided imagery and helpful suggestions providing soothing, rhythmical tones where the subject readily enters this hypnotic state of subconscious.

As the subject relaxes, the breathing becomes calm, the temperature goes down, the pulse rate slows, and the blood pressure falls. There may be signs of rapid eye movements (REM's,) and then the hypnotist attempts to discover the underlying causes of depression, or other disorders that have been suppressed. Despite rumors to the contrary, it is virtually impossible to hypnotize anyone against their will. No person under hypnosis can be made to do anything against what they consider to be wrong, or against their principles – if there were a threat, they would simply snap out of the trance and return to the waking state.

Rest assured – there is no such thing as someone becoming transfixed into a trance state. Speaking of rest, the worst thing that could happen is that the subject would fall asleep naturally, which would only be for a short duration, inevitably to awaken completely out of the trance. The best subjects are those who are imaginative enough to picture the ideas suggested by the hypnotherapist. Influenced greatly by the hypnotist's soothing words and guided imagery, such susceptible subjects often drift off into a relaxed dreamlike state, eventually reaching the **Subconscious Deeper Trance State.**

Although going into a trance is thought of as being asleep, this is a real misconception – the trance state is not much different than the normal daydream state. The only differences being that, with the eyes open or closed, self-hypnosis or autosuggestion may be delivered, or being that positive suggestions using guided imagery may be administered by a hypnotist, or hypnotherapist.

Before anesthetics became widespread in the middle 19th century, hypnosis had been commonly used in surgery. However, the use of hypnosis in America today is becoming increasingly popular, especially in surgery as an alternative to anesthetics, which can have unpleasant and sometimes dangerous side effects. Because it is so effective, hypnosis is increasingly being used to treat many disorders such as anxiety, stress, addiction, insomnia, and other psychosomatic complexes.

(continue)

__UNDERSTANDING HYPNOTHERAPY__ (continued)

As far as stage hypnotists go in America, law has restricted hypnotism used for entertainment purposes. The only hypnotist known to be doing well today is Paul McKenna, and the reason is because he knows the true value, as well as the benefits of hypnosis, whether on, or off stage. This highly creative approach to hypnotherapy provides an intellectual powerhouse, regarding mastery of the mind. More importantly, it initiates the total performance of the capabilities of the triune brain. Why should your client's dream of living a long and happy life continue to be illusive when it is well within their grasp?

__OF SPECIAL NOTE__

If you have concluded that you would treat persons by placing them into a trance state in order to renew their spirits, you would be right. All people are spiritual beings, whether having religious beliefs, or not. And since the spirit is supernatural in essence, it would follow that the mind should be penetrated on a subconscious level, rather than trying to communicate with its earth-based, conscious counterpart. Since the spirit is a supernatural state of mind it is best reached by bypassing the conscious state – thus allowing the therapist to go directly into the subconscious in order to enable reprogramming. This is because the conscious mind always tends to interfere due to its critical, skeptical, and other negative conditioning. But the subconscious is just part of what makes up our supernatural state.

Nearly all scientists, physicists, and psychologists (especially Carl Jung,) have come to agree that the mind is made up of genes handed down through time by our ancestors. That being the case, it should explain why going into the subconscious is so effective – because this was precisely where our minds took root and became formulated in the first place. Tapping into that source is the challenge and the secret to unlocking the true power of our mind, our subconscious mind. And since the subconscious rules our thoughts, this is definitely the place to begin the transformation process.

Anyone who wants to can benefit from hypnotherapy, except for those who are seriously mentally ill, very young children, persons with serious heart conditions, or those with uncontrolled epilepsy. Unless it is a typical hypnosis induction (such as giving up smoking, phobias such as fear of flying, confidence boosting, and the like,) it is always best to advise the potential candidate to consult their doctor, beforehand, so that organic medical problems can be ruled out ...EJL

CHAPTER TWO
2

FUNCTIONING
AS HYPNOTHERAPIST

---

2   HYPNOTHERAPIST
FUNCTION:

Autosuggestion became Emile Coue's doctrine during 1857-1926. He claimed that the hypnotist creates in the patient's subconscious an image of the desired effect, and that it is brought about, primarily, by the patient. Dr. Coue also claimed that each individual is a powerful hypnotist.

"Learn to cure yourself. You can do it. I have never cured anyone. This power is within you. Call on your mind for help. Make it the servant of your mental and physical well being. It will be present; it will heal you. You will be happy," he would say to his patients. He would also direct his patients to repeat the following affirmation twenty times, morning and evening:

"Every day, in every way, I get better and better."

CHAPTER TWO
2

FUNCTIONING
AS HYPNOTHERAPIST

HYPNOTHERAPIST:

While functioning as a hypnotherapist, preventing diseases from occurring, you are likely to add between ten and twenty years to many lives - including your own. By bombarding the subconscious, infiltrating it with new truths, hypnotherapy enables us the power to make changes for the better in our lives. The most effective way to instill belief is to bypass the conscious mind, which tends to edit, criticize, or restrict information from being processed. This where hypnotherapy plays an important part: through the use of the hypnotic trance it is possible to deliver positive messages directly into the subconscious where they become acknowledged without undo reasoning - hence, the process of transformation begins to take affect.

The hypnotherapist is a mental health practitioner who uses hypnosis to treat persons for mental, physical, or emotional disorders; a therapist who uses hypnosis to induce therapeutic healing to resolve psychological issues – hence, the function becomes that of a hypno-therapist. Through the Hypnotherapist, words will begin to paint images on the subconscious mind. These images will aid in mastering control over lives in creative and ideal ways through the process of hypnotherapy.

As the hypnotherapist, guided imagery and positive suggestions will begin to paint images on the subconscious mind. These images will aid in mastering control over lives in creative and ideal ways. The hypnotherapist's Function is to see that the subject becomes relaxed and focused. The intention is that you become capable of receiving suggestions and directions that will motivate you into taking complete control of your destiny. Since this book is about the function of the hypnotherapist we will be addressing the subject, or client. The client should be made aware that upon reaching the trance state they would not do anything to violate their own values. The fact is that they always have the power to terminate the hypnotic state at any time.

THE TRANCE ZONE HYPNOTHERAPY

Hypnotherapy is effective in discovering the full potential, as well as the depth and nature of the person being hypnotized, so that growth, self-esteem, and success may be achieved.   Through the hypnotherapist, words will paint images on the mind. These images will aid in mastering control over behavior in creative and ideal ways. During this process subjects will not become under anyone's control; rather, through unleashing the innate subconscious powers they will become enabled with the hypnotherapist's most powerful tool – namely hypnotherapy. In the state of hypnotherapy, the subconscious mind becomes fully accessible, processing two hundred million sensory messages every second. Conversely, in the conscious state, the mind is less than ten percent operational, processing only a handful of instructions at any given time.

Nearly all scientists, physicists, and psychologists (especially Carl Jung,) have come to agree that the mind is made up of genes handed down through time by our ancestors. The secret to tapping the depths of the mind is to go into the subconscious, where the true source of power rules. Since hypnotherapy works best in the state of relaxation, it is highly recommended that hypnotherapists predispose their clients to exercise, affirmations, and positive thinking, as well as having them listen to tranquil music.

The wonderful thing about hypnotherapy is that the nervous system cannot tell the difference between real and imagined experiences. By gaining access to the subconscious, the hypnotherapist can induce a trance and guide the subject into going anywhere, doing anything, or give the person permission to become anyone they wish. Just imagine: Functioning as a hypnotherapist, you can create an ideal reality in the client's mind, and actually have them feel, as well as experience all its benefits.   Creating and developing mental images is certainly a great way to sense what it's like to be successful, or what it feels like to be loved and wanted. In addition to the many wondrous musical sounds nature has to offer there are the sounds of bowls, drums, and the harmonica that can have a peaceful effect on the calming the mind.

Other tranquil sounds may come from waves, and such. In this hypnosis and hypnotherapy book you will learn how to unleash the power of the subconscious mind and change negative habits of thought and action into what you desire them to be. This is where, and how, you can begin reprogramming minds in order to utilize the brain's unfathomable resources.

THREE PREREQUISITES TO THE APPLICATION OF THE TRANCE ZONE HYPNOTHERAPY

DESIRE – Without desire going into the state of hypnosis, or transforming the mind will become difficult. Whatever it is you wish to accomplish with your subjects it must be applied with a **healthy attitude, and well-intended purpose**.

BELIEF – "***Whatever you can believe, you can conceive***," Robert Goddard once said. And he should know – he was one of the scientists who helped develop our first missile rockets. Not only should you believe in the process of self-hypnosis, but you must also have faith in the induction process when engaging the services of a hypnotist. Belief and trust go hand in hand when striving to accomplish anything. For hypnotherapy to work properly there must be a mutual feeling of trust between the subject and the hypnotist.

EXPECTATION – To **expect** is to anticipate the coming of something your subjects may desire. When subjects anticipate they muster up hope and believe that what you wish for will come to fruition. The preparation for your subjects, or patients, is **being willing, ready, and able to accept** what it is they desire to happen. Success can only be achieved through the expectation of positive results.

CONTEMPLATE THIS:

To *"Go Into" The Trance Zone* brings about an altered state of consciousness whereby, as if being some mystical power, the whole psyche shifts into an exaggerated state of positive exuberance. It is similar to that of *"the zone"* which athletes refer to when that inner force takes over and places the participant into a state whereby every movement seems effortless.

Tennis players and runners call this state *"the second wind"* where every challenge seems a breeze; every barrier becomes an invitation to a winning frame of mind. Remarkably, there is a surge of energy where everything falls into a state of euphoria referred to as the *"success zone."*

THE POWER OF HYPNOTHERAPY

As you strive to fulfill your dreams, you will come to realize that you alone are in complete control of your destiny.   In the state of hypnosis, the subconscious mind is fully accessible, with the entire brain processing one hundred million sensory messages every second. (Illustration 2-1)

Conversely, in the awakened state the conscious mind uses less than ten percent of the brain's potential, processing only a handful of information at any given time. (Illustration 2-2)

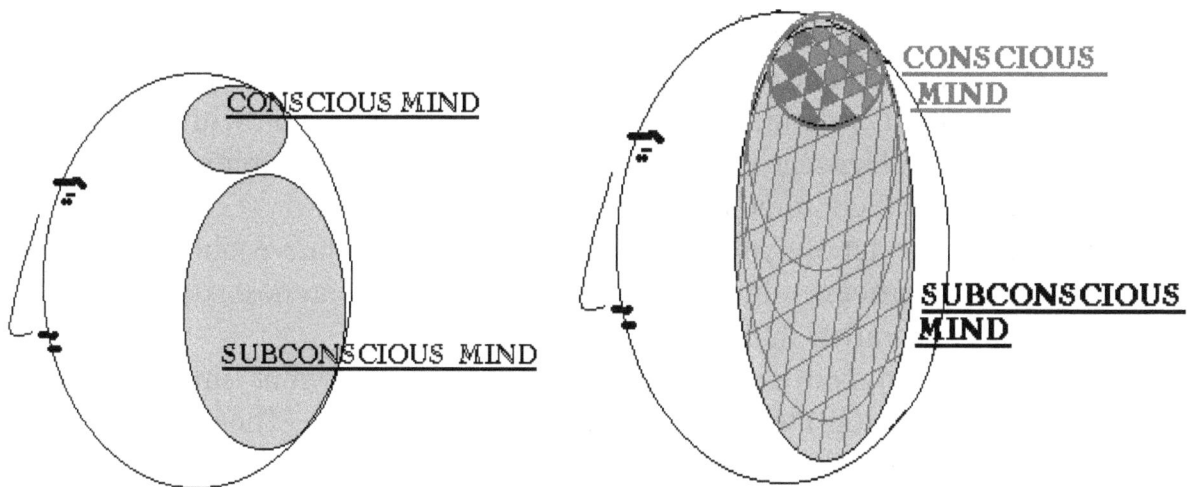

Illustration 2 -1 *(less than 10% of potential)* **Illustration 2 -2** *(fully accessible)*

Note: In the state of hypnosis, the subconscious mind is fully accessible, utilizing the maximum amount of the brain's potential – insomuch that it even takes control of the conscious mind.

Consider this statement from Carl Sagan, the legendary Professor of Astronomy and Space Sciences who suffered from a rare bone marrow disease, *"the subconscious possesses the incredible ability to process over a hundred million bits of information in a mere second."*

We teach by Precept, we teach by Habit,
we teach by Example . . . Aristotle.

HYPNOSIS DEFINED:
HYPNOTHERAPIST INDUCED HYPNOSIS (posthypnotic suggestion)

The word hypnosis comes from the Greek word, "hypnos," meaning sleep, to sleep, or to lull to sleep. In actuality, hypnosis is not of the sleep state, but rather of a trance-like daydream state, where the senses are awake and fully aware. If the subject does go to sleep, the hypnotic session is over – unless awakened.

Webster's New World Dictionary defines hypnosis as "a trance-like condition usually induced by another person, in which the subject is in a state of altered consciousness and responds, with certain limitations, to the suggestions of the hypnotist." It also defines hypnotize as "to spellbind." Mosby's Medical Dictionary defines hypnotism as "a trance-like state, resembling normal sleep, during which perception and memory are altered, resulting in greater susceptibility to suggestion." Another definition states: "hypnosis is relaxation with an agenda."

The American Heritage Dictionary defines the term, subliminal as "being below the threshold of conscious perception."

In essence, the act of hypnosis is really a highly meditative, subliminal, and sometimes psychic process – but it is more of a spiritual awareness, or trance induced dream state, rather than that of sleep.

In performing hypnosis, the subject cannot cause an arm or limb to become cataleptic (rigid like a log,) while the hypnotist is able do this. The reason for this has to do with the hypnotherapist's power over the subject, which poses this question: If the subjects are always in control of the session, how healthy is it to allow the hypnotist to take such control over their precious subconscious minds?

The answer is that the subject has a choice of turning the power over to the hypnotist, benefiting by years of professional experience, or of choosing not to undergo such an enriching process. While the subject can choose to practice and become an exceptional self-hypnotist, consideration must also be given to whether the benefits of using a professional outweigh one's own creative ability at mastering this complex phenomenon called hypnotherapy.

Then, of course, the subject can reason that the only control is through the self, and that no one has the power to overcome anyone else's mind. However, the subject should bear in mind that the hypnotherapist does not take control. The synergy derived from duality has tremendous credence, with much to be gained from the spiritual and chemical reactions, as well as the concerted interrelations between the hypnotherapist and the subject's subconscious mind.

(Note: **Posthypnotic Suggestions** are the messages, key words, or triggers induced by the hypnotist to the subject in the hypnotic state.)

SELF-HYPNOSIS DEFINED
SUBJECT INDUCED HYPNOSIS (autosuggestion)

Autosuggestions are the messages, or words induced by the subject to induce the self-hypnotic state, therein called self-hypnosis.

Webster's New World Dictionary refers self-hypnosis to autohypnosis and defines it as "The act of hypnotizing oneself or the state of being so hypnotized."

Actually, through **autosuggestion** the subject makes suggestions to the self, hence affecting the mind, thoughts, and bodily functions, thereby becoming hypnotized. When the subject performs hypnosis on the self, the process is called self-hypnosis or the act of **self-hypnotism**. **Self-hypnotic suggestion, self-hypnosis, or autosuggestion** is that state of hypnosis induced by the subject.

In performing self-hypnosis, the subject cannot cause an arm or limb to become cataleptic (rigid like a log,) while the hypnotist is able do this. While the subject can choose to practice and become an exceptional self-hypnotist, consideration must also be given to whether the benefits of using a professional outweigh one's own creative ability at mastering this complex phenomenon called hypnotherapy. Then, of course, the subject considering **self-hypnosis** can reason that the only control is through the self, and that no one has the power to overcome anyone else's mind. However, the subject should bear in mind that the hypnotherapist does not take control. The synergy derived from duality has tremendous credence, with much to be gained from the spiritual and chemical reactions, as well as the concerted interrelations between the hypnotherapist and the subject's subconscious mind.

THE INSIGHT OF MENTAL IMAGERY

No matter which aspect of thinking, the mastery of the mind begins with Mental Images. Every positive image brings a positive result. Every image brings to the fore its corresponding counterpart. Since every image brings a corresponding reaction, you can successfully influence the conscious mind through the subconscious mind. Our Mental Images, far more proficient than our thoughts, control our lives. Induce positive visualization to take root in your subconscious, and you can take charge – you can become master of your fate. You can obtain everything your heart desires.

In conjunction with Mental Images: since hypnotism produces organic responses, every negative thought must be counteracted by a positive thought. In this manner, the participant is able to become self-hypnotized, or be hypnotized into a life of success, gratification and joy. This is The Insight of Mental Imagery!

A GUIDE TO HYPNOSIS and HYPNOTHERAPY HEALING
Transformation, Transference, and *The Trance Zone*

Have you noticed that when things feel POSITIVE everything falls into place?
What about the correlation between nervous tension and relaxation?
How We Can Reverse Emotional Disorders and Alter Mental Illness?

Transformation: When one learns to acknowledge, accept, and then apply positive information, that person will begin to become transformed. This could feasibly happen physiologically, mentally, or spiritually, depending upon the subject matter, how it is presented, and who delivers the message. For example, if a person was to have been known as an alcoholic with hostile behavior then began attending AA meetings, and then later became noticeably respectable among his neighbors - that person could be described as having been transformed. Transformation through hypnotherapy can often be even more effective.

Transference: While a person's subconscious mental perception may produce negative effects it can also be that state of mind where everything seems possible. This is the state where a person's behavior patterns may become influenced through association. This could either happen earlier in life, or it may become introduced depending on new theories, or priorities developed later in life. An example of transference is how children become hooked on smoking, perhaps by admiring their peers, or by feeling a sense of bonding upon being accepted by their friends.

***The Trance Zone*:** This is that deep hypnotic state of hypnotherapy whereby a person becomes focused and guided into relaxing, mentally and physically. In spite of how most people view hypnosis, it is merely a state of mind where every part of the body becomes totally relaxed. It is that safe place where stress, fears, and anxieties become dissipated, or perhaps entirely alleviated. Any person may reach the state of hypnosis merely by closing their eyes, slowing the breathing, and counting down into that deep state of released tension. The hypnotherapist merely presents positive suggestions, or guided imagery in order to add to the deepening state of relaxation. After reaching the deep state of hypnosis, patients generally report that it felt like taking a short vacation. And, this is the very reason why hypnotherapy works: When a person becomes relaxed and unencumbered by negativity, that person is more likely to become influenced by positive suggestions. Then, through Transference, it becomes the responsibility of the hypnotherapist to see that information is delivered positively, and effectively in order to provide successful Transformation.

PREVENTIVE MEDICINE
Preventive Medicine, Nutrition And Disease.

The doctor of the future will give no medicine, but will interest his patients in the care of the human frame, in diet, and in the cause and Prevention of disease . . .
Thomas Edison

Nutrition Induces Healing, Prevents Disease, and Slows Inevitable Death!
How Is It Possible To Slow Down The Aging Process?

• *Riddle: Have you ever wondered why an apple, when left whole, lasts for weeks on end, yet, after being cut or bitten into, begins to rot in a matter of hours of being placed aside?*

• ***Think, my friend!***

Especially during these times of stress and environmental pollution, there are always effective ways to choose between quality of life, and the fatality of death. Once the concept of preventative medicine and the value of nutritional foods is understood, it may soon become evident you have been following the wrong regimen. But before blaming yourself, you must also realize that your mistake was perfectly normal - that it was the American way. You must also realize that right now is time to make a change.

CASE IN POINT: If you are the average person, you have been drinking orange juice out of the container because the label read "100% tropical orange juice. Bull! Not only is there no fresh orange juice, there are enough chemicals in a half-gallon container to induce a cold, virus, even fever. Yet, Americans wonder why they become overweight or become physically, and sometimes mentally ill. Yes, believe it or not: *What you do to the body, you do to the mind also.* Now, the premise is set. You get the idea here: *Fresh and natural,* is the key.

• **Answer to Riddle**: The reason the apple begins to spoil is because of oxidation: rancidness, decomposition, and deterioration. The sooner all foods in their natural state are eaten, the fresher, More Potent the Nutrients.

• *The best way to longevity is to prevent chronic disease from taking your life prematurely. It may be consoling to know that at least one in four people die from a disease that is largely preventable. Usually it is one of the Big Five - heart attacks, strokes, cancer, diabetes and Alzheimer's. According to what is known as the H factor, there are more than a hundred medical conditions that can be avoided by preventing the cells from aging. Your physiological makeup consists of well over ten trillion cells. Some cells live only a few days others for several months, and millions of immune cells live for years then die and become replaced . . . EJL*

PREVENTIVE MEDICINE (continued)

Illustration A: Drink fresh hand-squeezed orange juice. Here's how: After selecting an orange form the store wash it off immediately. After slicing it in half then squeezing out all the juice, you should eat the oozing, excess pulp. Squeezing the oranges by hand also aids in strengthening the fingers. It is important to wash the oranges because, in addition to pesticides, you may ingest the germs of the many people who have handled them before you.

Illustration B: Soy foods, such as tofu, are good for maintaining a healthy prostate. Diet sometimes plays a role in prostate cancer. Japanese men, for example, are said to have the lowest mortality rate from prostate cancer in the world. Eating raw slices of garlic and ginger 3 to 4 times a day will stimulate the immune system. Raisins, legumes, grapes, apples, including sesame, sunflower, flax, and pumpkin seeds are all natural foods that provide much needed vitamins, and minerals immediately into the blood stream. All these foods are attributed to slowing down the aging process.

EXAMPLES OF GOOD NUTRITION:

Illustration A: Always eat plenty of steamed vegetables. Here's how: Select about half-a-dozen fresh vegetables. Then wash them off and place them into a pan of water, but not touching the water. There are several ways to do this: Either place the vegetables into a Chinese bamboo steamer, or into the folding three-legged spiral, and let the water beneath come to slow boil - where they eventually become "steamed." When ready to eat, add some olive, and pumpkin oil to give it flavor.

Illustration B: In addition to drinking plenty of water, always eat plenty of leafy, green salads fortified with olive oil, tomatoes, olives, onions and sliced garlic. Make sure all foods are fresh, letting nothing become rancid. Get going! This information is intended to set the tone of what good nutrition is all about.

NOTE: Nerve cells, or neurons, in the brain communicate with one another by way of chemical substances called neurotransmitters (or electrochemical messengers). In one neuron, an electrical signal (or nerve impulse) causes the release of a neurotransmitter from its nerve terminal. A second neuron detects this neurotransmitter and responds by producing an electrical signal. This form of communication between two nerve cells is known as signal transduction. Over the last 30 years, Greengard and his colleagues have developed a general model, which provides a rational explanation, at the molecular and cellular levels, of the mechanism by which stimuli – both electrical and chemical – produce physiological responses in individual nerve cells.

For more information on this Nobel Prize winner visit the following website: (2000 Nobel Prize: http://www.rockefeller.edu/pubinfo/nobelpress.nr.php)

THE NECTAR OF THE GODS
WATER AND OXYGEN

Did you know that the very tap **WATER** you have been drinking day after day, year after year, has been recycling through the never-ending process of evaporation, cloud formation, and downpours for millions of years? Really, recycled **RAIN** has been providing us with our drinking water all this time! Just think of the possibility that we have been drinking the exact water that millions of others before us have already drunk.

Water is the best cell energizer and resuscitator. (Caffeine, by contrast, drains energy. In the brain cells, water generates energy, coffee only releases it for brief periods). Water is the best tissue detoxicant. It is the best diuretic. It is the best enhancer of enzyme function of energy, detoxification, digestive and neurotransmitter systems. It is the best antidote for acidotic stress.

Perhaps you also know that the very **OXYGEN** you have been indulging in, year after year, has been recycling through your lungs – a never-ending process of circulation for millions of years? Yes, your recycled **BREATH** has been providing us with our breathing capabilities all this time! Just think of possibility that we have been circulating the exact oxygen others before us have already consumed.

Oxygen is the main life force, the absolute source of energy that empowers every single motor function, from the circulatory system, to the pumping of the heart, to the most minimal physical and neurological activity. Being deprived of this vital force for more than six minutes could lead to sudden death.

Seeking Cures To Alleviating Disorders & Mental Illness
Edward J. Longo, Board Certified Member of the American Board of Hypnotherapy advocates the following guidelines:

The Criteria of Emotional Maturity

- ❖ Learn to function well under difficulty, to deal constructively with reality.
- ❖ Acquire the flexibility to adapt, adjust, and cope with change.
- ❖ Strive to become free of tension, alleviate aggression.
- ❖ Discover satisfaction in giving, rather than being intent in receiving.
- ❖ Seek harmony when intermingling, especially when relating to strangers.
- ❖ Practice sharing and helping, rather than hating thy neighbor.
- ❖ Always take the responsibility to express love, rather than to anger.

PART TWO

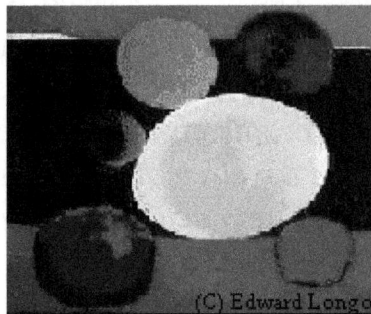

CHAPTER THREE
3

INTEGRATIVE MEDICINE
THE CONCEPT
BEHIND THIS BOOK

---

3 THE TRANCE ZONE HYPNOTHERAPY
THE CONCEPT:

At some deepened state, the adrenaline, metabolism, visual perception and intuition become increased inducing the elated feeling of being in "the groove." As this arousal state kicks in it becomes referred to as being "the zone," as many athletes have reported. This is the point whereby hypnotherapy then becomes organic in nature, and therefore everything seems to be functioning as if nothing could go wrong. Indeed, upon going into The Trance Zone Hypnotherapy it gives the feeling as though everything is going to wind up just right . . . EJL

CHAPTER THREE
3

**INTEGRATIVE
MEDICINE**
THE CONCEPT
BEHIND THIS BOOK

THE PSYCHOLOGY OF
THE TRANCE ZONE HYPNOTHERAPY

The Trance Zone Hypnotherapy connects to the life force, the true spirit of the soul within the physical body – in short it is the superlative energy of the subconscious mind. Indeed, this is the Majestic State of Mind. Upon reaching this subconscious state the feeling becomes one of splendor, as if subjected to a euphoric, majestic spell between the conscious mind and the spirit. It is that special, deepened trance state between the **Alpha** and **Theta** brain waves.

Being under the influence of hypnotherapy is to become charmed - it is tantamount to that of the Cobra, where the snake charmer casts a spell and causes it to respond from within a basket. Yet, the Cobra is not responding to the music, for it cannot hear - the snake is being charmed by the snake charmer's flute assimilating the movement of a pendant. Because of being highly focused on the flute, the Cobra cannot help but become hypnotized. This is the basis of the hypnotic trance, or hypnotism.

Hypnosis is not that of the sleep state, but of a false facsimile of sleep derived from the Greek God, "Hypnos," often associated with the hypnotic trance. This is the subconscious state where the mind in its entirety is most accessible. Because the conscious mind is judgmental and obstinate, it is restrictive compared to the subconscious. *The Trance Zone Hypnotherapy* is where the subconscious becomes empowered, free from criticism, detached from conscious intervention.

(continue)

THE PSYCHOLOGY OF
THE TRANCE ZONE HYPNOTHERAPY (continued)

When reaching the state of *The Trance Zone Hypnotherapy* many changes occur within the body. As the subject relaxes, the breathing becomes calm, the temperature goes down, the pulse rate slows, and the blood pressure falls. There may be signs of rapid eye movements as the mind shifts from consciousness to the subconscious state. The deeper the trance, the more unencumbered the body, and the more uninhibited the mind becomes.

At some deepened state, the adrenaline, metabolism, visual perception and intuition become increased inducing the elated feeling of being in the groove. As this arousal state kicks in it becomes referred to as being *"the zone,"* as many athletes have reported. This is the point whereby hypnotherapy then becomes organic in nature, and therefore everything seems to be functioning as nothing could go wrong. Indeed, upon going into *The Trance Zone Hypnotherapy* it gives the feeling as though everything is going to wind up just right.

At best, a state of euphoria will ensue, where mind, body and spirit feel so harmonious nothing becomes impossible to achieve. At worst, the state of total relaxation occurs, leaving the subject with the feeling that some kind of magic has been performed, some kind of vacation has been provided. In essence, all this is due to the natural release of endorphins and enkephalins.

The Trance Zone Hypnotherapy is that altered state of mind where the **Brain Waves** of the **Conscious** and **Subconscious Trance States** vibrate between 1 and 30 CPS. It is that unique place between the conscious and the sleep state, where the mind can reach its highest state of enchantment. It is that trance state of hypnosis, that place deep within us, where hallucination, amnesia, and fantasy take over the conscious mind, thereby subconsciously becoming realized as truth.

Asleep or awake, the mind's state of awareness is measured in brain waves from approximately 1 to 30 CPS, or **Cycles Per Second**.

(More information about the range of brain waves is provided below.)

STATES OF MIND
Brain Waves - Cycles Per Second (CPS)
(See **Illustration 3-1** below.)

The **Beta State** is reached when the mind is in its **conscious**, or **awakened** state where the vibrations measure from about14 CPS to as high as 30 CPS, or more, depending on anxiety, nervous tension, hysteria, etc.

The **Alpha State** is the beginning level of the hypnotic trance. It is reached when the brain waves become lowered from 13 CPS to 9 CPS at its deeper trance state.

The **Theta State** is reached when the brain waves become lowered 8 CPS, down to 4 CPS, or deeper, at its deepest trance state. The **Deep Theta State** is the deepest level of the hypnotic trance state.

The **Delta State** is reached when the brain waves become as low as 1 CPS at its deepest **sleep state**, increasing only to 3 CPS.

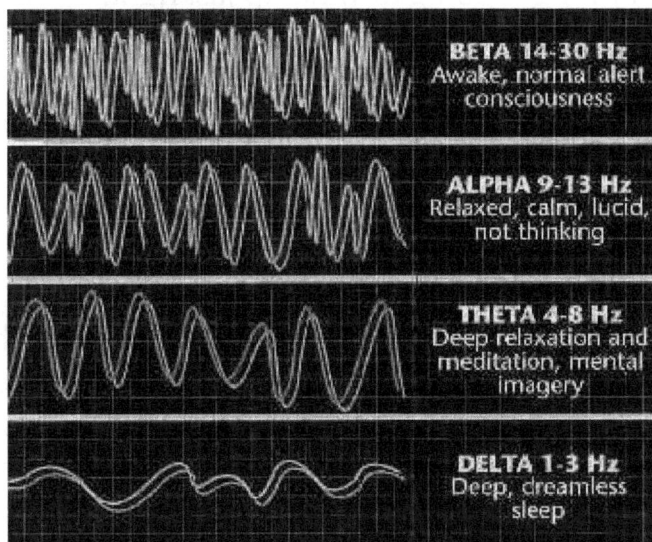

Illustration 3-1 - States of Mind – Brain Waves at Cycles Per Second

Note: Brain waves vibrating in the higher registers (above 30 CPS,) most likely would indicate hysteria, high anxiety, stress, or a virus invading the immune system. Rapid Eye Movement (REM) sometimes occurs during the Alpha state. This, however, is not an indication that a trance has been induced - it is merely the indication of a shift from the conscious to the subconscious trance state.

PSYCHOLOGICAL TOOLS
* EIGHT HYPNOTIC AIDS

Listed below, are descriptions of the psychological tools suggested in order to induce hypnosis in *The Trance Zone.* They are presented in the following order: **the hypnotic eye; eyes up to the eyebrows; deep yawn; inhale through the nose;** and **Hypnotic WORDS**. Other tools include **subliminal sounds; movement; and The Insight of Mental Imagery**. (Complete descriptions below:)

* The Hypnotic Eye

The posturing of the fingers has been commonly perceived as a sign indicating that everything is okay. Holding the hand in the air, indicating with the encircled thumb and forefinger has been widely used to represent many kinds of expressions, including perfection, to stress a point, or to demonstrate confidence. It has also been used to demonstrate security, or to express positive feelings. Regarding its role in The Trance Zone Hypnotherapy, this sign is used to trigger the connection to *"The Source."*

During hypnotherapy sessions the subject, or patient, is advised that, when forming this sign they are to refer to it as *"The Third Eye, the direct link to The Supernatural Spirit."* Ever since the discovery of that extreme, mystical power within the realm of The Trance Zone Hypnotherapy, I have become excited about its profound effectiveness. In realizing that the fingers subconsciously represent an extension of the subconscious inner spirit, or higher self, I have found the use of **"the hypnotic eye"** to be a very majestic way of inducing hypnotherapy.

(See **Illustration 3-2** below.)

Note: After conceptualizing this powerful hypnotic sign, it became surprising to see how many times people have used it on television to express themselves. At first, it seemed coincidental - but I don't really believe in coincidences. It is my firm belief that every idea becomes a universal consciousness - that people can become subconsciously influenced through some form of telepathy. So, it did not surprise me that placing the fingers together in this manner during hypnosis had caught on.

(continue)

PSYCHOLOGICAL TOOLS (continued)

As if designated for this purpose, it is interesting that **Alpha**, the subconscious, represented by the first finger, forms the position of dominance, while **Beta**, the conscious, represented by the thumb, constitutes the subordinate power. The leverage of **Alpha** becomes even more pronounced because of the **middle finger** representing the deep subconscious state of **Theta**, right behind it. What a coincidence that the last two fingers, the fourth finger and the pinkie, representing the varied sleep states of **Delta**, are farthest from the conscious state. The significance of this formation is quite mysterious, but I have found that there is no question regarding its unlimited effectiveness.

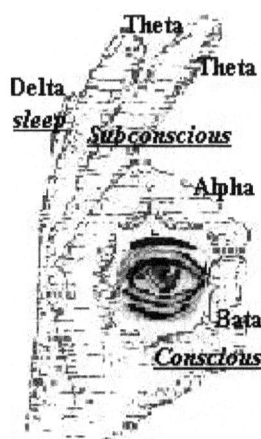

Illustration 3-2 – The Hypnotic Eye

As if designated for this purpose, it is interesting that **Alpha**, the subconscious, represented by the first finger, forms the position of dominance, while **Beta**, the conscious, represented by the thumb, constitutes the subordinate power. The leverage of **Alpha** becomes even more pronounced because of the **middle finger** representing the deep subconscious state of **Theta**, right behind it. What a coincidence that the last two fingers, the fourth finger and the pinkie, representing the varied sleep states of **Delta**, are farthest from the conscious state. The significance of this formation is quite mysterious, but I have found that there is no question regarding its unlimited effectiveness.

Forming "**the hypnotic eye**" is a powerful tool (see **Illustration 3-2** above), which aids in the process of hypnosis, in addition to providing an opening to supernatural intervention. Acting in concert with the **eyes up to the eyebrows, inhale through the nose,** and the **deep yawn,** placing the thumb and first finger together enables either the hypnotist or the subject to "Go Into" ***The Trance Zone.***

(continue)

PSYCHOLOGICAL TOOLS (continued)

One use of "**the hypnotic eye**" is to establish an association between the action of the fingers and lifting the **eyes up to the eyebrows**. This action serves as a trigger, transforming the psychosomatic/emotional conscious state into the subconscious trance state.

Other uses of "**the hypnotic eye**" are to gain a highly concentrated state of focus. This is accomplished by placing the fingers together as shown above and then by visualizing a supernatural third eye within the circle. The extraordinary powers of this action are explained in the examples given below.

Focusing to create a particular desire, result or need by concentrating on "**the hypnotic eye.**" For example: place the fingers together as in **Illustration 3-2** above and say the words, *I have so much money, I am financially independent.* To manifest a particular desire, focus on the center of "**the hypnotic eye**" while creating tension with the fingers and concentrating on the need. Focus on the Illustration below until you can associate it with the vision you have created in you mind. Then "Go Into" *The Trance Zone* and focus on positive visualization while keeping "**the hypnotic eye**" at your side.

PRACTICE EXERCISE: (See **Illustration 3-3** below.)

The **Illustration** below shows a number of ways to focus on quitting a bad habit, for example, **The Desire To Quit Smoking** is one way. You may concentrate on words, the pack of cigarettes, or the thought of quitting.

To augment this process, acquire a small crystal ball, place it inside the fingers that form "**the hypnotic eye**," and focus on attaining the desired result. Try to choose a clear, multifaceted crystal ball or one that is smooth; preferably blue, in color. Light up some frankincense during the ritual to produce even more effective results.

Whether in the need of quitting smoking, or wanting possessions, such as a Rolls Royce, love and romance, or financial gain, the principle of manifesting the result is the same. This works exceptionally well upon closing the eyes, going into hypnosis and imagining the ideal image, best dream, or desired outcome.

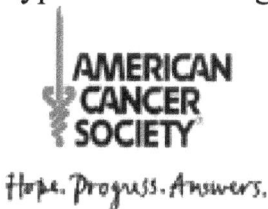

Quit Smoking

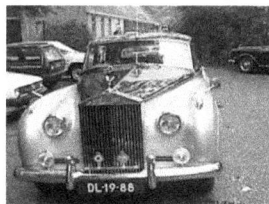

Possessions

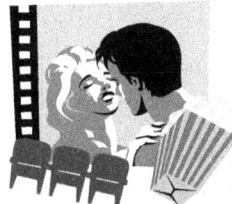

Love & Romance

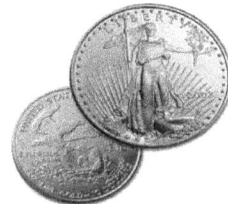

Financial Gain

Illustration 3-3

PSYCHOLOGICAL TOOLS (continued)

Focusing to induce instant hypnosis by placing "**the hypnotic eye**" above the subject's forehead.

PRACTICE EXERCISE:

As the hypnotherapist, have the subject stare at "**the hypnotic eye**" using either hand, and place it above the subject's forehead. Then have the subject lift the **eyes up to the eyebrows** and close them. Nearly automatically, this will induce the trance state. This should be reinforced by saying: *"This is how you 'Go Into' The Trance Zone."* (See **Illustration 3-2** above.)

PRACTICE EXERCISE:

As the hypnotherapist have the subject stare at "**the hypnotic eye**."
Then say aloud, *lift the* **eyes up to the eyebrows** *and close them.*
With either hand, form "**the hypnotic eye**" and place it above the subject's forehead. Then say aloud: *"This is how you 'Go Into'* **The Trance Zone**.*"*
(See **Illustration 3-2** above.)

Focusing to radiate love using "**the hypnotic eye**" over the subject's body to induce hypnosis for influencing love, as well as providing healing powers.

PRACTICE EXERCISE:

After placing "**the hypnotic eye**" near or over the subject's body, imagine the center having a laser beam whereby focusing intensifies the powers of personal magnetism, reciprocal love, and healing, as well as performing hypnotism.
(See **Illustration 3-2** above.)

Note: Focusing on "**the hypnotic eye**" is the key to unleashing the power of the subconscious mind. Whenever one calls upon this image hidden knowledge will be brought to light. Looking deeper and deeper within the spirit, one may draw wisdom from the depths of the subconscious mind. All knowledge is there for anyone who chooses to practice utilizing the connection to this Source - this Sacred Mantra. All channels of guidance become opened, especially intuitive and spiritual guidance. In this connected state, everything one could want to know shall become revealed. Everything becomes made clear; everything is exposed. Your will, as well as Thy will, will be done - and thus it is laid out before the participant. With practice, using the above procedure will not only improve the powers of hypnotherapy, but it will empower and enhance all aspects of mind, body and spirit. Whether the hypnotherapist, the subject, or the client, the most important thing to bear in mind is this: *What the subconscious mind can believe, the conscious mind can conceive.*   (continue)

PSYCHOLOGICAL TOOLS (continued)

Focusing to ward off evil forces by forming "**the hypnotic eye,**" and using the fingers to recite prayers. Note: By moving the thumb of the hand from the first finger and then back to the thumb, this becomes an extremely powerful method. The connection between the hand, fingers, and "**the hypnotic eye**" induces a very strong relationship with the protective, supernatural spirit.

PRACTICE EXERCISE:

Using the fingers as prayer beads is an ideal way to meditate, or to concentrate on relaxing. For an even greater effect read prayers aloud, as holy words become very powerful tools against evil influences.

An excellent way to use this method would be to go to the bible and read the verses of **Ephesians 6: 10 - 18.** (See **Illustration 3-5** below.)

Appropriately, I call the following set of prayers, *The Whole Armor of God.*

For the most effective results, be sure to follow these instructions to the letter: While placing the thumb and first finger together **recite verse 10** concentrating on the thumb; then **recite verse 11** while concentrating on the first finger.

Then continue, by placing the thumb and middle finger together, and then **recite verse 12** while concentrating on that middle finger. Then, placing the thumb and ring finger together **recite verse 13** while concentrating on that ring finger.

Then, placing the thumb and pinky together **recite verse 14** while concentrating on that pinky. Then, upon returning the thumb to the ring finger, **recite verse 15** while concentrating on that ring finger. Returning the thumb to the middle finger **recite verse 16** while concentrating on that middle finger.

Finally, returning the thumb to the first finger **recite verse 17** while concentrating on that same first finger; and **recite verse 18** while concentrating on the thumb.

For Use in memorizing details for total recall

After completing the following cycle of spiritual prayers, rest assured that you will be able to relax, no matter what the problem. Then, sit back and watch the demons vacate the premises!

(continue)

PSYCHOLOGICAL TOOLS (continued)

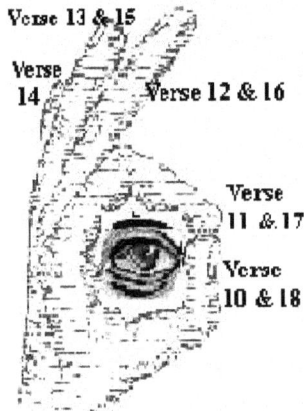

Illustration 3-5 - *Memorize the verses below by practicing the following sequence:*

Thumb & First Finger - (Concentrating on the Thumb):
Verse 10: "Finally, brethren be strong in the Lord and in the power of His Might."

Thumb & First Finger - (Concentrating on the First Finger):
Verse 11: "Put on the whole armor of God, that you may be able to stand against the wiles of the devil."

Thumb & Middle Finger - (Concentrating on the Middle Finger):
Verse 12: "For we wrestle not with flesh and blood, but against principalities, against powers, against rulers of darkness of this world, against spiritual wickedness in high places."

Thumb & Ring Finger - (Concentrating on the Ring Finger):
Verse 13: "Wherefore take unto you The Whole Armor of God, that you may be able to withstand in the evil day, and having done all to stand."

Thumb & Pinky Finger - (Concentrating on the Pinky Finger):
Verse 14: "Stand therefore, having your loins girt about with truth, and having on the breastplate of righteousness," (Notice that this finger is only touched once.)

Thumb & Ring Finger - (Concentrating on the Ring Finger):
Verse 15: "And your feet shod with the preparation of the Gospel of peace."

Thumb & Middle Finger - (Concentrating on the Middle Finger):
Verse 16: "Above all, taking the shield of faith, wherewith you shall be able to quench all the fiery darts of the wicked."

Thumb & First Finger - (Concentrating on the First Finger):
Verse 17: "And take the helmet of salvation, and the sword of the spirit, which is the word of God:"

Thumb & First Finger - (Concentrating on the Thumb):
Verse 18: "Praying always in the Spirit, and watching there for all Saints."

PSYCHOLOGICAL TOOLS (continued)

* eyes up to the eyebrows

Lifting the **eyes up to the eyebrows** and closing them triggers the conscious mind into the subconscious state. It is as if the eyes receive subconscious messages because they are parked within the synapse centers of the matrix of the brain.

* deep yawn

The reason for the **deep yawn** is, not only because it is contagious, but also because it aids in triggering the brain's subconscious activity. Yawning is a very effective way of relaxing both the body and mind in preparation to going into hypnosis.

* inhale through the nose

Focusing on **inhale through the nose** instructs the conscious mind to let go, allowing better transformation to the subconscious state. Since brain cells die at the rate of millions per second, this form of breathing enables the oxygen to replenish the brain cells at a more intensified rate. When breathing, think of breathing between the eyes. Sometimes, merely getting a person to smile during this time can make a great difference regarding attitude.

* Hypnotic WORDS

The keys to all hypnotic inductions are the **Hypnotic WORDS**, and the soothing, positive, reassuring manner in which they are executed. They have a specific energy and can be a very powerful influence on people, affecting their truths. **Hypnotic WORDS** delivered in the right rhythm and tones have an astonishing impact consciously. But when bypassed by the conscious mind, which restricts and edits, they become even more profound in the altered, subconscious state. Since you have been mesmerized through advertising, commercials, social interactions, and other means, negative messages have become imprinted within your subconscious. Transforming these self-defeating messages is the task of the hypnotherapist. The objective is to alter, reverse, or eradicate the condition so that you, or the subject, will become free of the psychologically damaging influences. While the mind, through repetitious bombardment, has accepted the notion that it may be prone to failure in all endeavors, the hypnotherapist can induce suggestions and, virtually, reverse the infliction. Through the hypnotherapist's voice, the **Hypnotic WORDS** can be delivered with such an infiltrating impact the subconscious mind could literally enable you to change the course of your life for the best. Practice speaking aloud, discovering the right timbre and cadence of your voice, and you will have discovered the foundation of a good hypnotist. (continue)

PSYCHOLOGICAL TOOLS (continued)

* subliminal sounds

In concert with the hypnotist's WORDS, *subliminal sounds,* serve equally well as they pacify the emotions; becoming formidable tools in penetrating the subconscious mind.   Subliminal sounds (or background sounds,) played or recorded during the hypnotic trance aid in inducing the hypnosis.   The sounds of a ticking clock or a metronome, musical instruments, animal calls, running water, ocean waves, and singing voices are all very effective means of soothing us and summoning the power of the subconscious mind. A great example of this is when a mother sings her child to sleep. The short, soothing song, classified as a "lullaby" has pacified many a baby to the point of falling asleep in its mother's arms -- a perfect example of a subconscious induction, and how it affects the mind. Other incidents, such as falling asleep during plays, operas, and movies are all reactions to subliminal inducements. Dozing off behind the wheel due to staring at the white line is another subliminal inducement -- a classic state of trance.

* Movement

Swinging pendants, bouncing balls, rocking motions, tapping fingers, and dancing - all can have a profound effect on the subconscious, positive, or negative.

* The Insight Of Mental Imagery

No matter which aspect of the mind, the mastery of it begins with your Mental Images. Every positive image brings a positive result. Every image brings to the fore its corresponding counterpart. Since every image brings a corresponding reaction, you can successfully influence the conscious mind through the power of the subconscious mind. *The Insight Of Mental Imagery*, far more proficient than our thoughts, controls our lives. Allow **Positive Visualization** to take root in your subconscious, and you can become master of your fate. You *can* obtain everything your heart desires. Since hypnotism produces organic responses, every negative thought must be counteracted by a positive thought. In this manner, you are bound to hypnotize yourself into a life of success, gratification and joy. The person who exercises and applies the **power of suggestion** through the subconscious mind becomes somewhat of a master. Having entertained the power of suggestion actually empowers almost all to achieve what is desired.

This is The Principle Rule of The Insight of Mental Imagery.

THE SECRET 7 GOLDEN RULES

The Trance Zone Hypnotherapy technique is extremely effective through its application of Hypnotic Inducements, Hypnosis Affirmations, and Majestic Trance Spells. This is a highly spiritual technique influencing dramatic changes for the good and best in life, where ideals, dreams, and heart's desires actually manifest into reality - even miracles.

The techniques and illustrations used in this book can become extremely beneficial regarding the informative and creative utilization of exercise, nutritional rehabilitation, and prayer. During your process of learning hypnotherapy remember to keep in mind **The Secret 7 Golden Rules** as outlined below.

1. If you like the way your life is going, great - enjoy it.

2. If you don't like the way certain things in your life are going, avoid them.

3. If you are not happy with certain things and cannot avoid them, change them.

4. Provided you are not content with the way certain things are and cannot avoid Change, or detach from them - then accept them.

5. To accept certain things you can try changing your point of view about them perhaps consider changing your mind.

6. Provided you cannot change your point of view about things, or change your mind about them, then draw upon the positive aspect of your subconscious to alter the situation according to your needs and desires.

7. Everything you are, or may become, is based on your **attitude**. Seek and incorporate the following **motivations** listed below in order to change your situation and you will be able to look forward to a full and complete life:

(continue)

THE SECRET 7 GOLDEN RULES (continued)
MOTIVATIONS

Purpose – With enough reasons to change your situation in life there must be something you wish to accomplish more than anything in the world. Then, by all means, find out what it is that you love to do and go for it with a passion!

Commitment – You must take a stand, whether it is something you believe in, or whether there is something you must do before you can move on - find out what that is, and stick to it, no matter what.

Focus – The key to success of every form is concentration. No matter what it is you wish to accomplish, learn to develop a direct plan of attack, a laser-beam focus, and hone in on it like a falcon going after its prey.

Passion – Find out what it is that makes your blood boil every time you think about it, then make it happen using every fiber of your being.

Interest – Money invested wisely produces interest. Invest wisely in yourself and investigate every avenue of endeavor until you can become excited about living a fulfilling and gratifying life - know and feel that you are worth it.

Drive – If your body was a vehicle and you wanted to make it from the East Coast to the West Coast, you would need to plan every detail to make sure you could reach your destination safely. Your mind is also a vehicle. With the proper strategy and a purposeful path, you should be able to reach your destination blindfolded. Living a gratifying, rewarding life takes that kind of determination.

Balance – If you are not able to develop a sound mind through prayer, music appreciation, exercise, health and proper nutrition, then you may be lacking in some physical or spiritual way. Other ways to develop mental balance and stability is change your pattern of sleep, environment, behavior, motivations, morals – even the way you dress and perceive yourself has an effect on your subconscious mind. Find every way possible to make all aspects of your life positive. "Know Thy self" helps – "Love Thy self" helps even more.

Prosperity – Seek this in every way, with one exception – do not focus on money as your idol, for you will only become subjected to "the root of all evil," which is Greed. Bear in mind that money is not the root of all evil – it is those unscrupulous, divisive extremes that people conjure up to acquire it.

Not only can *The Trance Zone Hypnotherapy* be used to advance your own growth but after learning these techniques the natural physician within will eventually become manifest. In fulfilling your potential to become a certified hypnotherapist, you will finally become qualified to perform hypnotherapy on future patients who are greatly in need of help.

POSITIVE VISUALIZATION:

The Ideal Way Of Bringing Ideas, Dreams, And Desires Into Reality

String Theory, Final Theory, and Theory of Everything – baloney! New Physics has taught us that energy can <u>never</u> be destroyed; that it simply changes form <u>eternally</u>. The very molecules our bodies have formed, the chemical make-up of our minds, and the atomic, electromagnetic energy of which our spirits are comprised, have always existed in one form or another. It would be foolish to think of individual energies as being cut off from each other. This is because there is, essentially, one energy source manifesting in multiple ways, functioning in a vast variety of forms. This Oneness that physicists are now discussing is what we have traditionally called the manifestation of God. Never doubt that when we intuitively tap into that universal energy, or consciousness, or collective subconscious, awesome supernatural power will commence to flow through our lives.

Science and Spirituality: New Physics Points To Cosmic Spirit

In the 1960s a cover story in *Time magazine* proclaimed: "God is dead," and had held science responsible for it. By the 1990s, people were questioning whether spirituality could promote health. The pendulum has now swung in the other direction. Ironically enough, it is the same science that once killed off the notion of God that is now strengthening humankind's belief in a "supreme power." the latest revelations in cosmology and quantum physics are fostering this paradigm shift.

At the University of California, Berkeley, an award-winning team of scientists has been conducting pre-clinical studies on aging. They discovered that by combining a natural, energy-boosting component (acetyl L-carnitine) with a powerful anti-oxidant (alpha lipoic acid) they could slow the cell aging process. Research has shown that an important factor in aging is the decay of the mitochondria – the organelles within the cell that convert amino acids, fatty acids and sugars into energy.

Note: The human DNA is a biological Internet and superior in many aspects to the artificial one. The latest Russian scientific research includes parapsychology healing called AIRES Matrix resonators. Other areas of research include phenomena such as clairvoyance, alternative medicine, intuition, remote viewing, and spontaneous acts of miraculous healing. Other areas consist of self- healing, affirmation techniques, the ability to see light auras, the mind's influence on weather patterns, and many other gifted attributes.

Reference: <u>Oneness Commitment</u> (www.experiencefestival.com)

CHAPTER FOUR
4

REACHING
THE DEEPEST LEVEL OF
HYPNOTHERAPY

---

4   HYPNOTHERAPY
INDUCTIONS:

The hypnotherapist hypnotizes the subject, whereby the subject becomes hypnotized through posthypnotic suggestions. When the hypnotherapist performs hypnosis on the subject it is called hypnotism.

Of <u>The Trance State Induction</u> I could reasonably say:
"Feed the subconscious mind enough optimism and it will flourish alive and well; feed it excessive negative, pessimistic thoughts and it will degenerate, inevitably to expire. I conclude that, for the hypnotherapist, the use of hypnosis is paramount in supplanting optimistic attitudes; it works equally well in providing treatment for disease and despair . . . EJL

CHAPTER FOUR
4

REACHING
THE DEEPEST LEVEL OF
HYPNOTHERAPY

HYPNOTHERAPIST'S INDUCTIONS
REACHING THE DEEPEST LEVEL

Penetrating The Subconscious Mind

Perhaps the most important thing to bear in mind regarding accessing the hypnotic state is this: In order to penetrate the subconscious mind, reaching a complete state of serenity allows the incoming message to take hold more effectively. The more the subject is able to relax, the longer positive suggestions will endure.

A Brief Entry to The Trance Zone Hypnotic State:
With either hand, form *"The Hypnotic Eye"* by placing the thumb and forefinger together, and place this hand at your side. This then becomes the eye to your subconscious mind which can be called upon any time you want to *"Go Into"* The Trance Zone hypnotic trance state. With the eyes closed and placed *"up to the eyebrows, "take in a deep yawn"* and focus on relaxing your breathing. Then recite: *This is how I go into the trance zone, where peace and tranquility allows me to enter a deep meditative state of mind.*

Entering into the trance state is quite a simple process because, after all, hypnosis is merely a state on focused relaxation. It is through this relaxed state that positive results can nearly always be ascertained. Because the conscious mind becomes by-passed, or disarmed, the subconscious readily accepts everything it receives as the TRUTH. When spiritually administered through hypnosis, positive suggestions manifest into REALITY through the supernatural energy delivered to the subconscious mind.

Note: Reaching the state of tranquility also serves to disarm the conscious mind, thus allowing the subconscious to override all unnecessary censoring. This is one of the reasons exercise is stressed so frequently within the context of this book.

TESTING THE TRANCE ZONE INDUCTION

To demonstrate the effectiveness of hypnosis, again form *"the hypnotic eye"* with both hands and interlock the centers, that is, the thumb and first finger of one hand encircling the thumb and first finger of the other. Now, lift the *"eyes up to the eyebrows"* and try to pull them apart while thinking, and speaking, *"I can not pull my fingers apart."* The fact is that you will never be able to pull them apart as long as you firmly commit to believing you cannot.

To prove this, continue thinking you cannot pull them apart, while saying, *"I can pull my fingers apart."* As long as you are thinking you cannot, you will not be able to pull them apart because your thought has generated a contrary, subliminal message to your subconscious. The principle is the same if you reverse the process. While thinking, *"I can pull my fingers apart,"* you will be able to – even though you say, *"I can not pull my fingers apart."*

The Conclusion: Irrefutably, the positive subconscious is the dominant power over the negative conscious mind)

THE TRANCE ZONE INDUCTION:
TO *"Go Into" The Trance Zone*

The Initial Procedure - (induced by the hypnotherapist)
To *"Go Into" The Trance Zone,* induce the hypnosis as follows:
First, have the subject form *"the hypnotic eye"* by placing the thumb and first finger together and place it at either side. Then, have the subject lift the *"eyes up to the eyebrows,"* close them, and give a *"deep yawn."*

Next have the subject recite: *This is how I "Go Into" The Trance Zone."* Now, instruct the subject to *"inhale through the nose"* and exhale while counting down from 30 by 2's, relaxing the body more and more while going into the hypnotic state. (Due to the many variations, counting down is optional.)

(This is how *The Trance Zone* is initially induced. The intention behind repeating this is to have it act as a posthypnotic suggestion, a subconscious trigger to *"Go Into"* the hypnotic trance more easily.)

Note: Generally, sentences appearing in *italics* throughout this manual represent the *voice*, or WORDS, of the subject or hypnotist. Both the WORDS of the SUBJECT and the WORDS of the HYPNOTIST are always shown in *italics*. The main difference between the dialog of the SUBJECT and the HYPNOTIST is that the subject's WORDS are always shown in the "first Person."

1ST INDUCTION TEST (with the subject sitting)
    HYPNOTHERAPIST:

Have the subject *"Go into"* <u>*The Trance Zone*</u>, as described previously, then continue with the hypnotic suggestions.

I'd like you to form "the hypnotic eye" and place your hand at your side. This is the eye to your subconscious, which puts you into <u>The Trance Zone</u>. Now, I'd like you to lift your "eyes up to the eyebrows" and, when you feel like it, close them. Keeping your eyes up take in a "deep yawn," and then recite: This is how I "Go Into" <u>The Trance Zone</u>.

In that wide opening to your subconscious, you are listening intently to my voice. Under hypnosis, you can speak to me if I ask you to. I'm now going to ask you to deepen your own hypnosis by remembering the order of the numbers when I count from 10 to 1 in this order: 10, 9, 8, 7, 6, 4, 3, 2, 1. I also ask you to say the words <u>deeper I go</u>, between my counts. By saying this you will go deeper into hypnosis 10, 9, 8, 7, 6, 4, 3, 2, 1. Good going. Now repeat the numbers as you just heard me count them. If you wish to add <u>deeper I go</u> with them, that's okay.

(This procedure tests the depth of the hypnotic state. If the subject remembers to leave out the 5, proceed with the hypnosis - if not, repeat the count down. Then proceed with the hypnosis using any of the inductions.)

2ND INDUCTION TEST (with the subject sitting)
    HYPNOTHERAPIST:

Have the subject *"Go into"* <u>*The Trance Zone*</u>, as described previously, then continue with the hypnotic suggestions.

I'd like you to form "the hypnotic eye" and place your hand at your side. This is the eye to your subconscious, which puts you into <u>The Trance Zone</u>. Now, I'd like you to lift your "eyes up to the eyebrows" and, when you feel like it, close them. Keeping your eyes up take in a "deep yawn," and then recite: This is how I "Go Into" <u>The Trance Zone</u>. In that wide opening to your subconscious, you are listening intently to my voice. As you are resting comfortably you will notice that your eyes are closed tight, very tight. They are stuck so tight you are not able to open them. In a moment I will ask you to try to open them - you will not be able to do so. You will find they are sealed tight - they are stuck firmly together. You may be able to manage the muscle groups around your eyes, but not your eyelids. No matter how hard you try, you will be unable to open your eyes. When I count down from 3 to zero, you will find it impossible to open your eyes and you will go deeper into hypnosis. 3 - Your eyelids are sealed tight, 2 - They are stuck tight, 1 - They are stuck firmly together, Zero. Try, but you are unable to open them. Stop trying.

(The procedure above provides an example of reaching the depth of the hypnotic state. If the subject becomes relaxed, proceed with the hypnosis - if not, repeat the process differently. Then proceed with the hypnosis.)

POSTHYPNOTIC SUGGESTIONS:

Posthypnotic Suggestions are the "CUES," messages, key words, or triggers induced by the hypnotherapist to the subject in the hypnotic state. The aim is to have them carry over to the awakened state. They are also used as a trigger to have the subject return to the hypnotic state.

For example, the hypnotherapist can give the subject a word, such as "**golden nugget**," under hypnosis, and upon being given that command in the awakened state, the subject will return to the hypnotic state. Also, snapping the fingers three times, while the subject repeats, "***I can do***" three times under hypnosis, can induce self-confidence when the command is executed in the awakened state. **Posthypnotic Suggestions** act as tools, in order to enable progressive treatment. In this instance, forming "**the hypnotic eye**" would enable the subject to rapidly "*Go Into*" *The Trance Zone* in subsequent sessions. Invariably, the subject's eyes will close very rapidly, inducing the trance.

Since all posthypnotic suggestions become effective when induced during the trance state, have the subject "*Go into*" *The Trance Zone*, and repeatedly give the subject the "trigger" phrase: *This is how you Go Into The Trance Zone.* After a few visits, the subject will easily go into hypnosis. Have the subject encircle the thumb and forefinger to form *"the hypnotic eye."* Then have the subject place the *"eyes up to the eyebrows,"* close them, and give *"deep yawn."* Then give the posthypnotic suggestion, (or "trigger") which will become the subconscious "cue" to go into the trance state.

HYPNOTHERAPIST:
This is how you "Go Into" The Trance Zone. Every time I give you this message, it will be easier for you to go into hypnosis. Now, with your fingers forming "the hypnotic eye," go into your trance and then go deeper into hypnosis.

Note: Posthypnotic suggestions can even work during self-hypnosis, executed by the subject. Self-hypnotic suggestion, self-hypnosis, or autosuggestion is that state of hypnosis induced solely by the subject.

Deepest Level   69

Influencing The Subconscious Mind

Suggestions such as: ***I will not think of an apple with a worm inside***, causes just the opposite affect. First, because ***I will not,*** relates to the future in a negative sense; the subconscious only acknowledges the present, and it acknowledges suggestions in a positive sense. Then, the words ***an apple with a worm inside,*** evokes a **vision** of an ***apple with a worm inside***. This is because the subconscious overlooks the negative term, ***not***.

The hypnotherapist, always looking on the brighter, positive side, would be wiser to choose to suggest: ***You are able to imagine an apple with its rosy colors***.

TYPICAL HYPNOTHERAPY INDUCTION

HYPNOTHERAPIST: (with the subject sitting or lying)

Have the subject *"Go into" The Trance Zone* as described below, then continue with the hypnotic suggestions.

I'd like you to form "the hypnotic eye" by placing the thumb and forefinger of either hand together, and place your hand at your side. This is the eye to your subconscious, which puts you into The Trance Zone. Now, I'd like you to lift your "eyes up to the eyebrows" and when you feel like it, let your eyelids close.

Keeping your eyes up take in a "deep yawn," and then recite: "This is how I "Go Into" The Trance Zone."

Good. In that wide opening to your subconscious, you are listening intently to my voice. Now, I'd like you to inhale through the nose and exhale through the mouth, while I count down from 12 by 2's, relaxing your body more and more while going into the hypnotic state. 12 . . . 10 . . . 8 . . . 6 . . . 4 . . . 2 . . . 0.

As you allow yourself to become free of tension, imagine yourself rising up into the sky where you become so high you become surrounded by enormous, white puffy clouds. Try to visualize yourself lying down right in the middle of one of those clouds with all the attributes of your present condition. Include your feelings, your attitude, and your present state of mind.

Picture yourself lying there with everything negative in your life - all the excess baggage, including, the headaches, tension, guilt, paranoia, illness, addiction to alcohol, drugs, or cigarettes, or any other agony you wish to get rid of. The important thing is to imagine unloading everything that bothers you as you become free from negativity. Acknowledge this being possible - see it all vanish. When I count from 1 to 5 you will remember everything that happened in your trance. Every part of you will feel better than ever before. 1 . . . 2 . . . you feel alert and refreshed, 3 . . . 4 . . . you are alert and alive and you will open your eyes feeling alert, refreshed and fully alive. 5 . . . open your eyes.

HYPNOTHERAPY INDUCTION - FOR INDUCING HOPE

HYPNOTHERAPIST: (with the subject lying down)

Have the subject "*Go into*" *The Trance Zone,* as described below then continue with the hypnotic suggestions. Note: During this process, it is highly suggested that you have some soft, relaxing music playing in the background.

I'd like you to form "the hypnotic eye" by placing your thumb and forefinger together, and place your hand at your side. This is the eye to your subconscious, which puts you into The Trance Zone.
Now, I'd like you to lift your "eyes up to the eyebrows" and when you feel like it, let your eyelids close. Keeping your eyes up take in a "deep yawn," and recite: "This is how I go into The Trance Zone."

In that wide opening to your subconscious, you are listening intently to my voice. I'd like you to inhale through the nose and exhale through the mouth while we count down together from 30 by 2's, relaxing your body more and more while going into your hypnotic trance. Okay, 30 . . . 28 . . . 26 . . . 24 . . . 22 . . . 20 . . . That's very good, your breathing is deep, relaxed. 18 . . . 16 . . . 14 . . . 12 . . . 10 . . . 8 . . . 6 . . . 4 . . . 2 . . . 0. That's very good. As you keep listening intently to my voice know that because of over-activity, troubles and regressive thoughts, the conscious mind tends to override the subconscious. In doing so, it tends stifle your free mind, interfering with your natural ability to go into the trance state. We are all capable of going into hypnosis because we do this naturally every day. To alleviate your problems, I'm going to ask that you go deeper into that wide opening to your subconscious where you feel safe, and unaffected by worldly influences. As you lie still, completely relaxed and tranquil, imagine rising above the earth and settling into a large, soft, white cloud. It is a moonlit night, and the cloud is completely illuminated, supporting your weight, holding you spellbound within its magnificent splendor.

Imagine being completely enveloped by the illumination of this cloud, as you become totally absorbed in the power of its pure whiteness. Within these surroundings, have this become your ideal place of serenity, of solitude, of comfort where you feel completely detached from your world. Here, you are completely protected, and devoid of all your problems. Here, is the place where you can experience total peace and total serenity. Now, in all your calmness in that wide opening to your subconscious, you are listening closely to all my words. Every moment you become better and better. You become calmer and calmer with each passing moment; and with each minute you feel more and more positive about yourself.   *(continue)*

HYPNOTHERAPIST: (continued)

As you listen intently to this message, you realize that all your faults, all your weaknesses, and all your failures have just become meaningless. What is now meaningful to you is that you enjoy life, a life that is so unique and so wonderful, you can now begin to appreciate it more and more.

From this moment forward, you will begin to appreciate your blessings. You will not only realize how great it is to be living, but you will come to appreciate your surroundings. Suddenly, you will appreciate the air you breathe, the trees you are privileged to see, and the flowers you able to smell. From this moment forward the foods you taste, and the wonderful music you hear will take on a new meaning. Right now, you can imagine all this, and you now feel your senses becoming aware, invigorating you while accepting that all of this is important to every aspect of your life.

As you keep listening to my words, you acknowledge that all is love, and that love becomes everything through living day by day in a positive fashion. Know that, even at this very moment, you feel a great appreciation of life, and that you are something more precious than you have ever imagined. Yes, you are not only precious to yourself - you are very precious to those around you. You see, because of this renewed you the world will have a greater chance of becoming a better place to live.

Now, as you leave that place and come down safely from that cloud, you arrive here with a renewed sense of life, a rejuvenated spirit, and a completely restored sense of hope. You feel completely relaxed and at peace with everything around you. As for your problems, they have become the least of you concerns. What you are concerned with, now, is how to live your life to its fullest, completely free of negativity and conflicting emotions. Because you have acknowledged being connected to this supernatural power your subconscious has accepted all this as fact. Know that you can rely on this source, this divine intervention as being permanent from this day forward.

When I count from 1 to 5 you will remember everything that happened during your trance. Know that every part of you will feel better than ever before. 1 . . . 2 . . . you feel wonderful and refreshed, 3 . . . 4 . . . you will open your eyes feeling alert, refreshed and fully alive. 5 . . . it's time to open your eyes.

Note: To see more examples of actual trance scripts performed by this expert hypnotherapist / psychotherapist, proceed to: Actual Scripts Performed On Clients.

HYPNOTHERAPY INDUCTION - FOR EMPOWERMENT

HYPNOTHERAPIST: *(with the subject sitting)*

Using the information provided so far, have the client *"Go Into"* <u>The Trance Zone</u> as described below and continue with the hypnotic suggestions.

I'd like you to form "the hypnotic eye" by placing the thumb and forefinger together, and place your hand at your side. This is the eye to your subconscious, which puts you into <u>The Trance Zone</u>. Now, I'd like you to lift your "eyes up to the eyebrows" and, when you feel like it, let your eyelids close. Keeping your eyes up take in a "deep yawn," and recite: "This is how I go into <u>The Trance Zone</u>." That's very good. In that wide opening to your subconscious, you are listening intently to my voice. Now, I'd like you to "inhale through the nose" and exhale through the mouth, while I count down from 12 by 2's, relaxing your body more and more while going into hypnosis. 12 . . . 10 . . . 8 . . . 6 . . . 4 . . . 2 . . . 0.

You are resting, calmly, relaxed, while your eyes are closed with your arms and legs are flexible. You are free of tension, nothing distracts you as you feel yourself being drawn along, breathing slowly, regularly. You are completely relaxed as you feel this wonderful peacefulness enveloping your being. In this state of peace you acknowledge that opening to your subconscious. This opening grows wider, more and more. My words are settling into your subconscious, are taking root there. I now offer the following empowerment suggestions: So far you have been using only a small fraction of your mind - your conscious mind. You have been using less then five percent of your true potential because of using only your conscious mind. Now, using the natural power of the subconscious, you are able to use more and more of your true power. Right now you have permission to use the total power of your subconscious mind. Every minute of every day your mind gets better and better in every positive way. Every minute of every day, your mind continues developing to its fullest potential - even now, it now has become better in every possible way.

When I count to five you will open your eyes feeling alert and refreshed. Every part of you will feel better than ever before. One, two . . . you feel alert and refreshed, three, four . . . you are alert and fully alive. Five . . . open your eyes.

(Note: Part of the hypnotherapist's obligation is to guide the subject into the trance state by offering helpful hypnotic suggestions, and by verbally painting colorful images, or guided imagery. Aside from experience and creative talent, the hypnotherapist's WORDS are, perhaps, the most powerful of all the tools. Do not become disappointed if it doesn't seem the client will experience the trance - even though it is very likely. Hypnotherapy does take lots of Practice, Patience and Persistence - the three P's of any successful endeavor.)

HYPNOTHERAPY POWER
IT BOILS DOWN TO THIS:

"Most people are skeptical about hypnotherapy because they don't understand it - the same way they fear everything they have never tried before. Once they come to understand and incorporate the power of the subconscious mind, even their most desirable dreams will manifest, as if by magic. Trying to accomplish the same feats by way of the conscious state could feasibly take a lifetime. In essence, people should be more skeptical of the limits of the conscious mind, rather than to fear the unlimited power of the subconscious mind. The subconscious mind is that place where all things become manifest into reality. The prerequisite is that one believes that all things are possible - and then allow the positive and mystifying powers of the supernatural take their course. Finally, they must come to realize that through the powers of the subconscious, <u>Nothing Is Really Impossible</u>."

Personal Messages From The Author / Founder
Mission Statement: "Inspire the injured spirit and you can dissipate any disease."

NOTE: Regarding the practice of The Trance Zone Hypnotherapy as a professional hypnotherapist, please have your clients be advised of the following information:

If you want things to go right close your eyes, form **"The Hypnotic Eye"** *and connect! You see - you don't have to do a thing except CONNECT to The Source. Hence, you allow the higher, supernatural power do all the work! I hope I have not wasted my time trying to get you to do this. I am telling you again: Commit to doing this wholeheartedly, and IT WILL WORK.*

You are being attacked by negativity - and since I can't get to you in person this is the next best thing. If you have not already done so, please TRY and experience the connection. Try to FEEL IT! Try to experience the Divine Intervention by focusing on the "EYE! Read the hypnosis manual, study the hypnotherapy certification book, use hypnosis tapes - but TRY to make the connection.

You have tried your way, now Connect MY WAY, and you WILL be provided with the right answer - NOT necessarily Your answer - but the Right answer.
Personal Empowerment Mantra: *"The Hypnotic Eye"*
Memorize the following mantra then practice using it. I guarantee it will work!
"This is The Hypnotic Eye, the eye to my subconscious, which is the link to the supernatural power." . . . EJL

5 Star Testimonials Given By Graduates

Hypnotherapy Certification ★ ★ ★ ★ ★
Certification through Mr. Longo's Hypnotherapy Course has empowered me to do just that. Through this remarkable course I have even qualified to become certified by the American Board of Hypnotherapy, (ABH) as a certified hypnotherapist. Edward Longo's concept is outstanding, and I recommend The Trance Zone Hypnotherapy Course to anyone who wants to learn to heal them selves, change negative behavioral patterns, or even start a rewarding career as a certified hypnotherapist. The Trance Zone Hypnosis Manual is the foundation to The Trance Zone Hypnotherapy Course . . . Robin E. Jones, TTZ Certified Hypnotherapist, Florida.

Hypnotherapy Certification ★ ★ ★ ★ ★
Greetings Ed. Just thought I'd share with you a recent success story. A patient presented me with "scraping trauma" whereby during meals, if metal touched metal, the plate, or a persons teeth, the patient would immediately suffer debilitating symptoms including: Headache bordering on Migraine, and begin feeling sick to her stomach to the point of having to leave the table. Using the methods taught in your course I promised her complete relief with a single hypnotherapy session, and wrote a short script to accomplish this. Obviously a function of a past trauma or series of them from much earlier in her life there were two different ways to go, either regress her and find the root, or the simpler approach of determining the triggers, symptoms and behavior and "reprogramming" her subconscious mind. I quickly wrote a short script using The Trance Zone induction and deepener and put her under and administered the suggestions. Immediately following the session we tested the Patient with Fork, Knife and Plate with complete success. In mere minutes I'd eased a life long debilitating condition that impacted not only the patient but her entire family. Your course made helping this woman a simple matter, as your approach and training follows a logical easy to use method, allowing the creation of scripts on demand for truly individualized therapy . . . Dr. Scott R. Senay, NJ

Hypnotherapy Certification ★ ★ ★ ★ ★
Although I had been working as a creative dancer I always thought I could become an intuitive healer. During my introduction to Edward Longo at one of his seminars I became so highly connected it was as though I had become reborn. The Trance Zone hypnosis manual gave me an experience that was truly enlightening, as well as rewarding. Thankfully, after confiding in this gentle man I made the decision, and commitment to take his course on hypnotherapy. I am happy to report that I am now a proud graduate of his school. Not surprisingly, Mr. Longo has always offered me his undivided attention, and complete support. He has definitely provided me with empowerment and freedom of The Spirit. This testimonial is one way of my thanking him . . . Jose Luis Jorge, certification #53104-HT, New York, NY

PART THREE

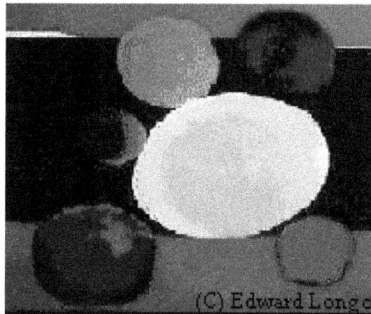

CHAPTER FIVE
5

REPROGRAMMING
THE SUBCONSCIOUS MIND

---

5   REPROGRAMMING
& PROGRAMMING:

Negative thoughts cause pessimistic behavior patterns, just as pessimistic behavior patterns cause negative thoughts. People say, "sticks and stones shall break your bones, but names shall never hurt you.'"

Well, words can stick in your head; thoughts can stick in your mind. Negative things your parents, your friends, your enemies, and even total strangers have told you can become etched in the subconscious mind.

Like a recording, it plays, on and on, whether you are aware of it, or not. Things you wouldn't dream of thinking consciously can be sitting there undermining your thoughts, sabotaging your very ideals. The consequences can result in inner conflicts, turmoil and, sometimes, utter confusion.

Whether being a victim of temptation, alcoholism, smoking, or gambling, reprogramming the mind can alter these addictive, habitual behaviors. Indeed, hypnotherapy can alter these, as well as erroneous thought patterns, disorders, or negative personality traits.

. . . EJL

CHAPTER FIVE
5

REPROGRAMMING
THE SUBCONSCIOUS MIND

ALTERING THE BELIEF SYSTEM
THE MIND CAN ACTUALLY ALTER THE BRAIN!

According to psychiatrist Jeffrey Schwartz in a Newsweek article on February 26 1996, "The mind can change the brain." During the month of February, Dr. Schwartz and four UCLA colleagues reported in the Archives of General Psychiatry that the mind could be at least as powerful as medicine when it comes to remodeling the brain. Behavioral modification, (altering the way a person behaves,) and cognitive therapy, (altering the way a person thinks,) can alter the biology of their brains.

It is true that a leopard cannot change its spots – just as a person is not able to change the color of their skin. But as human beings we can adjust our thinking, which in turn may <u>alter our behavior</u> - which could lead to a change in our personality. Inevitably, some persons are capable of becoming subject to positive physiological, or psychological transformation regarding characteristics, identities, mannerisms, dispositions, or individual personality traits. Actors do this all the time. In order to induce a positive message into the subconscious the old message must be removed. In essence, the undesirable, old message is not automatically erased by the new message – it is nullified when inducing the desired, positive message.

Holding The Elephant Captive

Our minds, including our thoughts, can hold us captive. Because of certain conditioning our beliefs can become set, depriving us of all hope, of ever attempting to change our ways. Conditioning can go both ways - it can either hold us captive, or it can release us from our bondage. One way to become released from bondage is to practice repetition so positive the mind will come to believe it as being the truth. Positive repetitions, faithfully practiced, will eventually come to be accepted by the mind and become manifest into reality. For an example of such conditioning consider the circus elephant. When wild elephants are first captured in Africa they are placed in a holding pen with an impenetrable fence and held there for a certain period of time. This is the beginning of "brainwashing," whereby the elephant's behavior becomes modified. When they are subsequently sent to the circus environment they are shackled to the ground by one leg for long periods. Now considerably tamed, the only movement they are able to make is within the confines allocated by the length of the chain tied to a wooden stake.

In time, they grow accustomed to their limitations, accepting that they cannot break loose from the chain that held them for so long. Through repetition, they come to believe they can never escape their bondage. Weighing in at several tons it is obvious to anyone that with a simple tug the elephant could uproot the stake and be off and running. But these elephants do not know this – they have become conditioned to believe that freedom is not possible, so eventually, they give up trying. And so, we too, tend to give up when things seem fruitless – when we cannot seem to break away from the chain that binds us. That chain can be broken; the chain that holds us down is our belief system, or more appropriately, our conscious mind. And the way it can be broken is, not by brainwashing, but by brain conditioning, sending positive suggestions directly to the subconscious mind through the power of hypnosis.

Negative thoughts cause pessimistic behavior patterns, just as pessimistic behavior patterns cause negative thoughts. People say, "sticks and stones shall break your bones, but names shall never hurt you." Well, words can stick in your head; thoughts can stick in your mind. Negative things your parents, your friends, your enemies, and even total strangers have told you can become etched in the subconscious mind. Like a recording, it replays at the weakest moments, sitting there waiting for the opportunity to strike. Things you wouldn't dream of thinking consciously can be sitting there undermining your thoughts, sabotaging your very ideals. The consequences can result in inner conflicts, turmoil, utter confusion and oftentimes, mental illness.   (continue)

Holding The Elephant Captive (continued)

Very much like the elephant, we too tend to give up when things seem hopeless – when we cannot seem to break away from the chain that binds us. That chain can be broken; the chain that holds us down is our belief system. Our bondage is actually expressed through the conscious state of mind. The best way that chain can be broken is not by brainwashing, but by brain conditioning. The good news is that freedom from bondage, or negativity, can be accomplished by accepting positive suggestions through the use of hypnosis and hypnotherapy.

Keys To Making Positive Changes – Four Princilples:

The **first principle:** In attempting to alter negative behavior realize that we are all creatures of habit. Since positive habits are far more beneficial than bad habits, the key is to initiate a positive habit strong enough to overcome the unwanted habit. This can be accomplished by **developing new patterns**, or by selecting a habit so effective and enjoyable that it acts to disarm, or overpower the undesirable bad habit.

The **second principle:** In order to affect a change "**rename**" the habit. For instance, regarding being addicted to cigarettes say, "I am really having a nicotine urge," rather than "I am having nicotine fit." (Verbalizing the truth sometimes makes the best medicine.)

The **third principle:** Provided the case is true, "**attribute**" the urge to a biochemical imbalance in the brain, and begin developing new patterns. (Admitting that the problem is chemical, rather than having a mental weakness, is closer to the truth, relieving unnecessary guilt. Then the impetus to change becomes easier.)

The **fourth principle:** In order to affect change "**refocus**" on some positive, constructive activity for fifteen minutes. This engages another part of the brain and alters the brain circuits that initially caused them to become stuck.

(In **developing new patterns** by "**renaming**," "**attributing**," and "**refocusing**" it is possible that the mind may be able to rewire the neural synapses that cause phobias, depression, or other debilitating disorders.)

PHYCHOLOGICAL ADJUSTMENT

Everyone develops habits, but most are positive, while many others are negative. The problems rise when our negative, or bad, habits control us – for they begin inducing demoralizing and abusive, self-defeating traits. Whether falling into patterns of negative conditioning, or self-destruction – reprogramming our thoughts can be successfully used to alter the defeatist personality. Through the application of Psychological Adjustment, the hypnotherapist is now able learn how to actually alter thought patterns, as well as personality traits. Transformation can be achieved by practicing the following:

Altering Thought Patterns

Without realizing it, people become so set in their way of thinking they never realize that changing their attitude could be an option. Sometimes it is possible to influence a subject's thought process by making direct, helpful suggestions during the hypnotherapy induction.

In the following example of a hypnosis trance script, the desired message serves to replace the negative, fixated message:

Your old feelings, attitudes and fixations about smoking have now been dismissed. They are now erased and extracted from your subconscious, so that they are replaced only by positive confirmations. As far as your health and your breathing, you now have but one healthy desire - and that is that you breathe clean, fresh air, rather than saturating your system with smoke. Throughout the day, you shall breathe only the fresh air given to you naturally, unencumbered by needing to have filthy objects placed in your mouth, while stupidly sucking on them. From now on, your desire to smoke has been altered so that the need is unnecessary. Your need to smoke, as well as the nicotine craving, is now eliminated.

Continue below for more on Psychological Adjustment.

(continue)

PHYCHOLOGICAL ADJUSTMENT (continued)

Altering Thought Patterns (continued)

Alter The Thought
Just when you think it is time to quit; that's the ideal time to begin.
Why not learn to become the head, instead of the tail.

Change The Focus
To break a negative bad habit, replace it with a positive good habit.
Life is hard by the yard; by the inch it's a cinch.

Build Self-confidence
Everything is all right now; everything will continue to be all right.
First, love yourself then you will be able to give love, as well as accept it.

Instill Motivation
To accomplish a goal, find a believable reason for it.
Acknowledging that life is but a breath is seeing a life more precious.

Induce Belief
What the subconscious mind can believe, the mind can conceive.
Know that changing the word can't to can do, all things become possible.

Create Hope
With the new beginnings of today, come the opportunities of tomorrow.
Every minute of every hour, you are better because of having this power.

Develop A Positive Attitude
You cannot decrease your age, but you can behave as being younger.
Everything you do is right, because it comes from the best within you.

PHYSIOLOGICAL ADJUSTMENT
Whether being a victim of temptation, alcoholism, smoking, or gambling, reprogramming the mind can alter these addictive, habitual behaviors. Indeed, hypnotherapy can alter behaviors, as well as erroneous thought patterns, disorders, or negative personality traits. Through the application of Physiological Adjustment, you will learn how to alter personality traits of **The Spirit, The Mind**, and **The Body**. To begin adjusting your life consider the following:

ALTERING PERSONALITY TRAITS
PHYSIOLOGICAL ADJUSTMENT can be readily be achieved through Unleashing The Power Of The Subconscious; The Subconscious Genie Within; and Accessing The Fountain Of Energy. See full descriptions below.

UNLEASHING THE POWER OF THE SUBCONSCIOUS:
THE SPIRIT - the internal and external subconscious energy

The Spirit is the all-knowing, all encompassing power of our being, our very soul. Feed your spirit prayer and affirmations and you will receive inspirational thoughts, and countless blessings. Through **The Spirit**, you can not only learn to develop inspirationally, but you can learn to grow emotionally as well – in important ways, such as compassion, understanding and, most of all, love. When you learn to live in **The Spirit**, you will become entirely alive, living within the powers of your subconscious, supernatural mind.

THE SUBCONSCIOUS GENIE WITHIN
THE MIND - the conscious and supernatural subconscious energy

The Mind, as the fundamental organ of human life, comes complete with its supernatural compliment, called the subconscious. Together, they form the most complete organism of all the species on earth. Through this unique formulation of organs, glands, circulatory and nervous systems there is nothing that can't be accomplished. With all its brain cells, synapses, and intuitiveness, this combination has conquered every obstacle in order to reign supreme. With that being said, it should mean that every individual has the same chance of becoming effective. However, not all individuals are able to make use of this amazing facility. Through bypassing the conscious mind and going into the hypnotic state, you have the opportunity of altering your mind so that you can attain whatever it is you desire. And, when it comes down to bad habits, you will not have a great struggle with quitting smoking, or other negative addictions. All this will make more sense as you gain more experience and begin to know your self as a perfect and complete human being. Finally, as you regain your self-esteem you will feel all those negative gremlins fading by the wayside.

ACCESSING THE FOUNTAIN OF ENERGY
THE BODY - the internal chemical energy

The Body is the fountain from which we draw our natural source of energy. Because the energy provided by our body is so accessible, we expend it foolishly, making ill use of its astonishing power. In addition to mental and spiritual inspiration, we must keep it supplied with nutrition and exercise. Feed the body the proper nutrition and it will keep up the pace; refurbish it with exercise and it will beget the stimulation necessary to instill determination, as well as endurance. The following induction will aid in activating the endocrine glands, which cause the body to become relaxed, receptive and supple.

PERFORMING SELF-HYPNOSIS INDUCTIONS
SELF-HYPNOSIS PROCEDURE

Below is the **Self-hypnosis** trance procedure that is, typically, required in order to "*Go Into*" *The Trance Zone*. With the understanding that the trance script should be taped in the "first person," rather than being memorized, follow the instruction below to experience what it may be like to enter the trance state.

The inductions, as illustrated, are examples of the use of self-hypnosis. Whether the hypnotherapist, or the client, taping hypnotic scripts is an extremely effective way to unleash the power of the subconscious mind. After taping the following induction lie back, "*Go Into*" *The Trance Zone*, and listen to your own words until satisfactory results are achieved.

Tip: Hypnotism takes a lot of Practice, Patience and Persistence.
These three P's can be applied to any successful endeavor.

EXAMPLE OF A SELF-HYPNOSIS INDUCTION
SUBJECT INDUCED SELF-HYPNOSIS: (self-hypnotic autosuggestion)

Using the information you have so far, become seated comfortably and "*Go Into*" *The Trance Zone*. You can do this by memorizing the words below, or by first taping and then listening to it with full concentration. Imagine everything as vividly as possible. Do not become disappointed if it doesn't seem like you went into a trance – even though it is most likely you will do so.

SUBJECT: (self-hypnotic trance induction)

The image I have formed of "the hypnotic eye" is the key to unleashing the power of my subconscious mind. Whenever I call upon this image, hidden knowledge will be brought to light. As I look deeper and deeper within my spirit, I draw wisdom from the depths of my subconscious mind.

All knowledge is there for me. All channels of guidance are opened to me, especially spiritual guidance. Everything I want to know is revealed to me. Everything is made clear; everything is exposed. My will, as well as Thy Will, will be done – and thus all is laid out before me.

Note: Brief as this may seem, some persons will be able to go right into the trance state. The best way to gain this remarkable uplifting experience is to simply proceed without skepticism, or any doubt that this is actually possible.

ANOTHER A SELF-HYPNOSIS INDUCTION
SUBJECT INDUCED SELF-HYPNOSIS: (self-hypnotic autosuggestion)
Self-hypnotic Induction for Empowerment:

First, form "**the hypnotic eye**" by placing the thumb and forefinger of either hand together, and place it at your side. This is the eye to your subconscious. Then, lift your **eyes up to the eyebrows**, close them, and give a **deep yawn**.

SUBJECT ("*Go Into*" *The Trance Zone as follows:*)

This is how I "Go Into" The Trance Zone, where only good things happen. While I begin counting down from 12 by 2's until reaching zero, I inhale through the nose, and exhale through the mouth, relaxing the body more and more. I now count down with 12 . . . 10 . . . 8 . . . 6 . . . 4 . . . 2 . . . 0.

In that wide opening to my subconscious, I am listening intently to my voice. I am resting, calm, relaxed, my eyes are closed and my arms and legs are flexible. I am free of tension, nothing distracts me as I feel myself being drawn along, breathing slowly, regularly. I am completely relaxed as I feel this wonderful peacefulness enveloping my being.

In this state of peace I acknowledge that opening to my subconscious. This opening grows wider, more and more. My words are settling into my subconscious, are taking root there. I now submit to the following commands: So far I have been using only a small fraction of my mind – my conscious mind. I have been using less then five percent of my true potential because of using only my conscious mind. Now, using the natural power of the subconscious, I am able to use more and more of my true power. Right now I have permission to use the total power of my subconscious mind. Every minute of every day my mind gets better and better in every positive way. Every minute of every day, my mind continues developing to its fullest potential. Even now, it now has become better in every possible way.

When I count from one to five I will open my eyes feeling alert, refreshed and alive. One, two . . . I'm feeling alert and refreshed. Three . . . Every part of me will feel better than ever before. Four . . . I am alert and fully alive. Five . . . Feeling better, I now open my eyes.

Note: Again, <u>never,</u> during <u>any stage</u> of the hypnotic trance, is there any danger of not being able to "*Come Out*" of *The Trance Zone*. At worst, the subject will merely take a short nap and wake up naturally, feeling <u>completely normal</u>.

At no time will the subject, or patient, remain under the hypnotist's power. This is true even during hypnosis because the hypnotist merely acts as a guide, providing helpful, positive suggestions.

SAMPLE PRERECORDED PRACTICE TAPE:

The inductions shown below are examples of the use of self-hypnosis. Whether the hypnotherapist, or the client, taping hypnotic scripts is an extremely effective way to unleash the power of the subconscious mind. After taping the following induction lie back, "Go Into" *The Trance Zone,* and listen to your own words until satisfactory results are achieved.

For the purpose of using any of the hypnotherapist's inductions for self-hypnosis, be sure to change the wording to the "first person." The following illustration is an example of this. Imaginative variations of this illustration can be used to alter situations, resolve problems, and alleviate pain and sickness. Other creative variations can aid in achieving practically anything you desire.) Generally, sentences appearing in *italics* throughout this manual represent the voice, or WORDS, of the subject or hypnotist.

Both the WORDS of the SUBJECT, and the WORDS of the HYPNOTHERAPIST are always shown in *italics*. The main difference between the dialog of the SUBJECT and the HYPNOTHERAPIST is that the subject's WORDS are always shown in the "first person.")

Self-hypnotic Induction for Empowerment:

I understand that, due to the conflicts between my accountability and accomplishments, tension builds up causing much discomfort and despair – even disease. To alleviate these pressures, I begin by stretching all my fingers open wide. As I continue stretching my fingers, I open my mouth very wide and give a deep yawn. Even more, I stretch my fingers and stretch my jaws open wider. Taking another deep yawn, I close my fists then stretch my fingers. Again, I close my fists and stretch my fingers.

Now I relax all my muscles and take deep breaths as if allowing the oxygen to flow into the muscles of my jaw, shoulders, hands, legs and feet. I focus on this deep breathing until I feel tingling in different parts of my body. I really feel this happening. I feel the oxygen rejuvenating my body and spirit, replenishing my stamina. My entire body feels loose and my mind is so clear I feel all the stress leaving my being.

As I go into a deep state of hypnosis, I imagine going into an even deeper hypnotic trance. Using my imagination, I find the words to put my body in such a hypnotic trance, everything I can imagine, becomes possible. I see this, feel this, and will experience the results of my wishes, desires, and most magnificent dreams as they manifest into actual truth.

Note: The trance state is not a sleep state, but rather the completely relaxed state prior to going into the normal sleep state. The worse thing the subject could do is fall asleep while being hypnotized by the hypnotherapist, albeit taking a short nap and then awakening automatically within a short period. In some cases the hypnotherapist may prevent the subject from dozing off by adding words like: *Although you are deep into hypnosis you are focused, and fully aware of your surroundings.*

If sleep <u>does</u> occur, the session may have to be terminated.

There are several ways the trance may be terminated when administering hypnotherapy: It could either be terminated by counting upwards from 1 to 5, as demonstrated below, or it may occur naturally by the subject falling asleep. Either way, there is absolutely no danger, or any reason to worry about anyone ever coming out of the trance state – it is just not possible.

In order to *"Come Out"* of the trance, merely stop the session by opening your eyes. Counting from one to five is an excellent way to execute coming out of a self-hypnotic trance because it conditions you to becoming alert at the end of a session. If you happen to fall asleep that is okay too – you will awaken automatically, most likely retaining the messages in your subconscious. The reason it is best to stay aware during the trance state is to ensure that the subconscious does receive the messages. During any session, the subject always has the control to interrupt the trance at any time. If need be, the hypnotherapist may also choose various *"Come Out"* methods of terminating the trance.

Information Regarding Dreaming
Dream Fulfillment During Sleep – (see Majestic Trance Spells)

"The standard practice regarding dreams is to attempt to interpret them <u>after</u> they have occurred. However, to my surprise, I have discovered that if a person would set up a <u>Dream Fulfillment</u> request prior to going to sleep, that request would become actualized during the dream state. Then, upon awakening, the person would be able to recall, and experience everything the dream revealed. The request could be as simple as asking for a solution to a specific problem, or asking to live an experience that would bring a certain kind of fulfillment; sexual or financial gratification, for example. As you can imagine, this technique could produce richly rewarding results, having a remarkable, positive effect on one's welfare and self-esteem. Why not "Go into" a trance and discover the Genie within you. Whether calling upon your spirit-guide, visionary, mediator, or a God – Ask, Seek, Knock and You Shall Find." . . . EJL

CHAPTER SIX
6

ACTUAL SCRIPTS
PERFORMED ON PATIENTS

---

6   HYPNOTHERAPY SCRIPTS
APPLICATION:

Hypnotherapy Testimonial: *In the fall of 2000, I received some very helpful therapy through hypnosis sessions with Edward J. Longo. A short period later I received more progressive therapy while I studied the Hypnotherapy Course using the techniques based on his hypnosis manual called The Trance Zone.*

In addition to receiving my Certification through The Trance Zone Hypnotherapy Course I soon became certified by the American Board of Hypnotherapy (ABH) as a Certified Hypnotherapist. Since this training was so thorough, I was pleased when I was able to receive my valid Certificate Number #0907 without needing any additional training, or testing.

Jennifer Maslowsky, New York

CHAPTER SIX
6

ACTUAL SCRIPTS
PERFORMED ON PATIENTS

APPLICATION OF ACTUAL SCRIPTS
With Typical Examples

Hypnotherapy is still being widely practiced by psychiatrists, surgeons, doctors, and hypnotherapists alike, to treat disease. Because its effect is organic, hypnotherapy is truly a marvel of mind over mind. When used properly, it can be used as a tool to investigate past lives, probe into the problems of the psyche, and even traverse and envision what the future may have in store. The practice of hypnosis to enhance hypnotherapy is not a mere mental procedure - it has turned out to become a supernatural phenomenon that continues to behoove the average person, even to this day. Becoming hypnotized to overcome issues is definitely the wave of the future, where more and more people want to grow intellectually - psychologically, as well as physiologically. Finally, health, wealth, and the pursuit of happiness can be achieved by all who dare to become involved in one of the most revolutionary forms of treatment of the 21st century.

Although the above is by no means the only testimonial regarding my hypnotherapy sessions, Jennifer's testimony had an influence on my decision to make my hypnosis trance scripts more formidable. And, my main reason for this was that I had come to the realization that many persons, including clients, needed to know there was this profound hypnotherapy course available.

One of my most recent scripts was developed specifically for the purpose of giving short hypnosis sessions at my seminar at the New Life Expo at the New Yorker Hotel, in New York. I have included the actual trance script below.

The reading / delivery time should take approximately fifteen minutes.

Subconscious Power Trance
Short Version, with the Purple Aura

HYPNOTHERAPIST (have the patient *"Go Into"* The Trance Zone, as follows:)

I'd like you to form "the hypnotic eye" by placing the thumb and forefinger of either hand together, and place your hand at your side. This is the eye to your subconscious, which puts you into The Trance Zone. Now, I'd like you to lift your "eyes up to the eyebrows" and, when you feel like it, let your eyelids close. Keeping your eyes up take in a " deep yawn" and recite: "This is how I go into The Trance Zone."

Very good . . . That is how you "Go Into" The Trance Zone, where only good things happen. Now, I'd like you to "inhale through the nose" and exhale through the mouth while "counting down."

In that wide opening to your subconscious, you are listening intently to my voice. Please note that it is important to focus on the hypnotic eye with the three fingers extended. Use of the hypnotic eye will be helpful in having it serve as a tool. With practice this will become your source of personal self-esteem, your positive secret weapon. Your arms and legs are flexible, relaxed.

As we count down from 12 by 2's, continue breathing evenly, inhaling through your nose and exhaling through your mouth. When I say the number 12, take in a deep breath and begin counting down aloud. 12, 10, 8 . . . With each breath you sink deeper into a relaxed state of mind. 6, 4 . . . the lower the number the deeper you go into hypnosis. 2 . . . Zero. The deeper you go into hypnosis you go even deeper into hypnosis.

As you continue to listen to my voice just allow yourself to become open minded and completely open to my directions, positive suggestions, and guided imagery. Soon, these words will open your doorway to becoming transformed in an extremely powerful way. It is very important to note that rhythmic breathing is also used as a tool for going deeper into hypnosis. The calmer the rhythm established during this hypnosis session, the deeper the hypnotic state will become. So, in addition to focusing on the hypnotic eye, please focus on deep, relaxed breathing throughout this session.

Know that you are connected to the source that will provide you with all the security, self-confidence, and emotional assuredness you will ever need to make positive changes permanently. Right now hardly anything distracts you. Hardly anything will interfere with you going deeper into hypnosis. Only positive changes are going to take place. Only good things are going to happen as your mind becomes clear.

(continue)

Subconscious Power Trance (continued)

Your mind is free of all tension, free of all problems. You welcome this sense of freedom and well being that relieves stress from head to foot. Feel this wonderful relaxation as you experience the looseness and weightlessness of your body. Sinking deeper and deeper. <u>Now let your fingers loosen.</u>

Imagine every part of your body becoming so relaxed it seems like jelly. Each time you inhale think of the oxygen as being a purple purifying vapor coming into your spirit, cleansing you of all your impurities, of all your diseases. Now, imagine this purple vapor transforming into a purple aura surrounding your being. And now imagine this purple aura becoming a powerful enabling aura. Every time you breathe in, allow your purple aura to accumulate more positive energy. Focusing on your purple aura becoming more splendid visualize it as becoming your own spiritual steam. It is now the most wonderful feeling you have felt in a long time. In your subconscious, know that as these powerful words do their work, you will have become free from every emotional hurt. You will sense the relief of every injury, of every negative influence that has had an effect on you.

As you experience this special empowerment, know that you have become transformed. As you continue to focus on your purple aura, know that you are being protected from the influence of all harmful, or negative forces. Allow this imaginary aura relieving every pain, every stressful condition, every restrictive feeling in you body. Allow your aura to balance your entire nervous system, your complete immune system as you focus on allowing your mind to come to complete rest. You are free of all worry, free of all tension as you drift off into your hypnotic trance. Deeper and deeper you go into this deep trance state; deeper and deeper you go into hypnosis. The deeper you go into hypnosis, the deeper you go into this hypnotic state.

My words have an especially powerful influence on the neuro-psychological system within you. The beautiful words and special tones of my voice have been orchestrated to help stimulate your body's entire healing mechanism. These special words act as a powerful medicine to your complete mental system. These hypnotic words are being registered in your subconscious, right down to the complex activity of your nerves. These hypnotic sounds of my voice are actually performing healing, harmony and coordination within your entire body.

Your entire nervous system is adjusting to my positive words, allowing your mind to become completely whole, magnificently balanced. Let your breathing assist you into hypnosis.

(continue)

Subconscious Power Trance (continued)

Each time you inhale imagine receiving renewed vitality from the source of life that surrounds us - the universal energy which nourishes the plants and trees, which holds the birds in flight, and which blows the winds from the four corners of the earth. Each time you exhale remind yourself that you are also emptying away all disease, nervous disorders and feelings of negativity.
Continue feeling empowered as you experience Unleashing Your Subconscious Power.

Let the realization of these images sink into your being while focusing on your purple aura. Reassure yourself that you are not only breathing to retain life, you are breathing to live life, and to live life more abundantly. Remember that you are breathing to benefit your body, spirit and brain, as well as improving your character. Positively accept the fact that every lungful of oxygen is helping to enrich your spirit as well as your physiology, your entire personality. Feel and experience yourself becoming more confident, more filled with self-esteem. You can think of this as spiritual steam.

In your subconscious, you know you are completely able to fulfill these objectives. The true nature of your mind is that it wants to be healthy; it wants to be mentally sound. In that unique portion of your brain, there is a healing mechanism that is able to repair and regenerate itself. Your mind needs to feel successful; it strives to maintain a state of balance where every cell can function at its optimum performance. You know that your subconscious is able to do this, for it is the ultimate supernatural power. Deep down, you know that it knows what to do, and how to provide you with spiritual empowerment, instinctively. This is something that will stay with you even after you come out of this deep trance.

Right now I'd like you to focus on trusting your empowerment. The solution, the magic key to accepting all this permanently, is to focus. Focus on the relaxed muscles, and the purple aura you are imagining now. Resolve right now to keep your muscles relaxed, rather than tense and restricted. Resolve in agreement with your subconscious mind to have all unnecessary tension become a thing of the past. Resolve to have your stress, your anxieties and all you unfounded fears become completely resolved. Imagine having all negativity dissipate allowing you to finally become free from bondage. And now, in your own mind, truly accept the fact that your subconscious mind has agreed to handle this task. Have this renewed energy cover your entire body as you imagine it transforming into a dynamic, confidence-building, purple aura.

(continue)

Subconscious Power Trance (continued)

This powerful, relaxing energy overwhelms you to the point you feel a tremendous confidence in yourself. Right now, I'd like you to visualize yourself as being completely empowered, magnificently transformed. Your mind is free of all worry, free of all stress, and daily problems. Feel and experience this wonderful sensation. Imagine your inner physician as being part of your colorful purple aura, protecting you. Imagine this feeling as energy coming from your inner physician as it permeates throughout your body. You know you are capable of adjusting to this positive transformation, this new adjustment that is allowing you to become whole.

You know deep down in your subconscious that you are able to cope with any situation. Yes, you are now able to cope with any uncomfortable situation that causes unnecessary tension because you know this power is within you. When you come out of this very deep trance, there will be complete relaxation. You will experience complete relief from all unnecessary pain and anxiety. You will feel completely relaxed feeling relieved of any discomfort and stress, relieved of all unnecessary nervous tension, or pain. In your subconscious, know that you have become more and more relieved of every emotional hurt, of any mental disorders. You will sense the relief of every injury that has had a lasting effect on you.

This all-empowering, positive mode you are now able to relate to, is called The Trance Zone. Your subconscious has adjusted to my positive words, and will acknowledge and process everything that has been said. From now on, you will accept the fact that this remarkable, supernatural power is being bestowed upon you. To enforce your belief in this higher power, your subconscious has acknowledged all this and will remember everything as a fact.

Know that the beauty of inner growth is that it can be an endlessly enjoyable adventure. Remember that self-examination leads to self-insight. And self-insight leads to freedom of negative behavior patterns. In that safe place, deep within the darkest shadows of you mind, this supernatural process has already taken place.

As I slowly begin to count from 1 to 5, you will become better and better upon each count. 1 . . . You are feeling terrific knowing that you have finally been transformed. 2 . . . You remember everything that happened during this trance state. 3 . . . You feel happy having your positive personality. 4 . . . You are totally relaxed, fully aware, and feeling empowered. 5 . . . You are awake and feeling ten times better than ever before. Finally, you are healthy, alert, and fully alive. It's time to open your eyes.

APPLICATION OF ACTUAL SCRIPTS (continued)

THE TRANCE ZONE – THE INITIAL INDUCTION

The following has been repeated so that the Hypnotherapist could develop more expertise regarding the initial induction in order to "Go Into" The Trance Zone.

The Hypnotic Eye Technique (with the subject sitting or lying)
TO "GO INTO" THE TRANCE ZONE
HYPNOTHERAPIST (have the patient *"Go Into"* The Trance Zone, as follows:)

I'd like you to form the hypnotic eye by placing the thumb and forefinger of either hand together, and place your hand at your side. This is the eye to your subconscious, which puts you into The Trance Zone. Now, I'd like you to lift your eyes up to the eyebrows and, when you feel like it, let your eyelids close. Keeping your eyes up take in a deep yawn and recite: "This is how I go into The Trance Zone."

Very good -- that is how you "Go Into" The Trance Zone, where only good things happen. In that wide opening to your subconscious, you are listening intently to my voice. Your arms and legs are flexible, relaxed. Please note that it is important to focus on the hypnotic eye with the three fingers extended. Use of the hypnotic eye will be helpful in having it serve as a tool. With practice this will become your source of personal self-esteem, your positive secret weapon.

In that wide opening to your subconscious, you are listening intently to my voice. Please note that it is important to focus on the hypnotic eye with the three fingers extended. Use of the hypnotic eye will be helpful in having it serve as a tool. With practice this will become your source of personal self-esteem, your positive secret weapon. Your arms and legs are flexible, relaxed.

As we count down from 30 by 2's, continue breathing evenly, inhaling etc.

Continue with the hypnotic suggestions.

(Shown below is how *The Trance Zone* typical induction was initially induced. The intention behind repeating this is to have it become effective as a posthypnotic suggestion, the subconscious trigger to *"Go Into"* the hypnotic trance more easily.)

APPLICATION OF ACTUAL SCRIPTS (continued)

The Trance Zone Hypnotherapy – Typical Induction
TO "GO INTO" THE TRANCE ZONE
EXAMPLE:
HYPNOTHERAPIST (have the patient "*Go Into*" *The Trance Zone*, as follows:)
I'd like you to form the hypnotic eye by placing the thumb and forefinger of either hand together, and place your hand at your side. This is the eye to your subconscious, which puts you into The Trance Zone. Now, I'd like you to lift your eyes up to the eyebrows and, when you feel like it, let your eyelids close. Keeping your eyes up take in a deep yawn and recite: "This is how I go into The Trance Zone."

Very good . . . That is how you Go Into The Trance Zone, where only good things happen. Now, I'd like you to "inhale through the nose" and exhale through the mouth while "counting down." As we count down together from 30 by 2's, continue breathing evenly, repeating after me. Inhale after each count, and exhale slowly.

Let's begin . . . 30, 28, 26, 24, 22, continue counting down slowly. That's good, breathe slowly and calmly. Exhale as we keep counting . . . 20, 18, 16 . . . Just let your body relax more and more each time. That's right, inhale through your nose. Exhale as we keep counting . . . 14 . . . 12 . . . 10 . . . the deeper you go into hypnosis, the lower you sink into the center of the earth. 8 . . . 6 . . . 4 . . . 2 . . . Zero.

Proceed *with the hypnotherapy session by inducing various positive suggestions, and creative, guided imagery.*

Continue with The Trance Zone Hypnotherapy Induction below.
(The average patient hypnosis session should take approximately 30 minutes.)

APPLICATION OF ACTUAL SCRIPTS (continued)

Supernatural Power – Custom Tape, or CD (with the Purple Aura)
THE SECRET WEAPON INDUCTION
HYPNOTHERAPIST (have the patient "*Go Into*" *The Trance Zone,* as follows:)

I'd like you to form the hypnotic eye by placing the thumb and forefinger of either hand together, and place your hand at your side. This is the eye to your subconscious, which puts you into The Trance Zone. Now, I'd like you to lift your eyes up to the eyebrows and, when you feel like it, let your eyelids close. Keeping your eyes up take in a deep yawn, and recite: "This is how I go into The Trance Zone."

Very good -- that is how you Go Into The Trance Zone, where only good things happen. In that wide opening to your subconscious, you are listening intently to my voice. Your arms and legs are flexible, relaxed.

As we count down from 30 by 2's, continue breathing evenly, inhaling through your nose and exhaling through your mouth. When I say the number 30, take in a deep breath and count down. 30, 28, 26, 24 . . . With each breath you sink deeper into a relaxed state of mind. 22, 20, 18, 16 . . . the lower the number the deeper you go into hypnosis. Just let yourself go . . . 14 . . . 12 . . . 10 . . . the deeper you go into hypnosis, the lower you sink into the center of the earth. 8 . . . 6 . . . 4 . . . 2 . . . Zero.

Please note that it is important to focus on the hypnotic eye with the three fingers extended. Keep concentrating on this until you hear me say it seems like jelly. After practicing and forming the hypnotic eye while listening to this tape, remember to recite the following mantra many times throughout the week. Recite it with me now, or just listen to my voice and know it is your secret weapon.

This is the hypnotic eye, the eye to my subconscious, which is the direct link to the supernatural power. Use of the hypnotic eye will be helpful in having it serve as a tool. With practice this will become your source of personal self-esteem, your positive secret weapon. As you continue to listen to my voice just allow yourself to become open minded and completely open to my directions, positive suggestions, and guided imagery. Soon, these words will open your doorway to becoming completely transformed in an extremely powerful way.

It is very important to note that rhythmic breathing is also used as a tool for going deeper into hypnosis. The calmer the rhythm established during this hypnosis session, the deeper the hypnotic state will become. So, in addition to focusing on the hypnotic eye, please focus on deep, relaxed breathing throughout this session.   (continue)

Supernatural Power (continued)

The following will be a way of unleashing your subconscious power. Let every tense muscle relax. . . Let total relaxation happen. Right now hardly anything distracts you. Hardly anything will interfere with you going deeper into hypnosis. Only positive changes are going to take place. Only good things are going to happen as your mind becomes clear. Your mind is free of all tension, free of all problems. You rejoice in this sense of freedom and well being that relieves stress from head to foot. Feel this wonderful relaxation, which spreads more and more rejuvenating your entire body. Experience the looseness and weightlessness of your body as you feel yourself sinking deeper.

You have an opening to the subconscious -- wider and wider this opening has become. Your subconscious is registering all my words. The gentle words of my voice are being deeply engraved there as you listen intently to my suggestions. You are listening very intently as I proceed to empower your positive state of mind. Listen closely to these words as I say them to you: You feel peaceful; you feel very quiet emotionally. You feel calm physically, and you enjoy the peace, the quiet, and the secure feeling that permeates within your being. You readily accept this sense of security as becoming part of your personality

You are lying comfortably with your eyes still closed tight. Your arms are flexible, relaxed. Now concentrating on being loose and free, keep taking in deep breaths through your nose, exhaling through your mouth. Let your entire body relax while lying in this secure, comfortable position. As you continue to do this, think of the incoming oxygen as an elixir, a magic potion that cleanses you inside and out. Now think of this magic potion as a self-confidence potion entering your lungs. Allow this potion to fill you with such confidence that you feel it becoming part of your character. Have this feeling of self-confidence become abundant within you. This is something you can hold with you even after you arise from this trance, this deep trance you are entering into, deeper and deeper. Going deeper, and even deeper.

Now, breathing in deeply, take in full breaths as if you can picture the oxygen filling your lungs. As you continue to breathe deeply, imagine the oxygen as a magic healing vapor. The deeper you breathe, the deeper this healing vapor circulates into your entire body. The more oxygen you take in, the more you feel the effect of its subconscious powers. Visualize a clear picture of this supernatural vapor going into your lungs and circulating throughout your nervous system. Begin to think of this vapor as being purple in color. Now think of this color purple as being your special spiritual color. Let your breathing assist you into hypnosis. Inhaling through the nose allow your diaphragm to fill up with this vapor.

Supernatural Power (continued)

Imagine every part of your body becoming so relaxed it seems like jelly. Now relax your fingers and go deeper into hypnosis. Allow this imaginary vapor relieving every pain, every stressful condition, every restrictive feeling in you body. Allow this vapor to balance your entire nervous system, your complete immune system as you focus on allowing your mind to come to complete rest. You are free of all worry, free of all tension as you drift off into your hypnotic trance. Deeper and deeper you go into this deep trance state; deeper and deeper you go into hypnosis. The deeper you go into hypnosis, the deeper you go into this hypnotic state. Deeper and deeper, you drift off into your beautiful, restful hypnotic trance.

My words have an especially powerful influence on the neuro-psychological system within you. The beautiful words and special tones of my voice have been orchestrated to help stimulate your body's entire healing mechanism. These special words act as a powerful medicine to your complete mental system. These hypnotic words are being registered in your subconscious, right down to the complex activity of your nerves. These hypnotic sounds of my voice are actually performing healing, harmony and coordination within your entire body.

Your entire nervous system is adjusting to my positive words, allowing your mind to become completely whole, completely balanced. Let your breathing assist you into hypnosis. Inhaling through the nose think of your diaphragm, including your lungs, filling up with purple oxygen. Then exhaling through the mouth, keep a relaxed rhythm going as you listen to these positive words. Each time you inhale imagine receiving renewed vitality from the source of life that surrounds us - the universal energy which nourishes the plants and trees, which holds the birds in flight, and which blows the winds from the four corners of the earth. Each time you exhale remind yourself that you are also emptying away all disease and nervous disorders. Emptying away all ailments, depression, and feelings of negativity. This is the kind of power you are enabled to tap into. Still remaining aware of your surroundings without going to sleep, continue to go deeper into hypnosis. Continue feeling empowered as you experience Unleashing Your Subconscious Power.

Being that you may tend to be a workaholic on and off the job learn to leave your professional work details at work. One way to do this is to make notations on a special pad and leave that pad in a gone fishing drawer, or compartment. Another way to stop thinking about work after work is to wear a hat as your professional thinking cap while working, and then make sure to take it off when your day is done.

(continue)

Supernatural Power (continued)

Still another way to leave your work at work is to think of yourself as developing self-confidence each time you detach from performing your duties after work. Know that positive thinking will come about when you realize you are not getting paid this kind of overtime. Eventually, it will become evident that dwelling on issues after work is nonproductive. Remember that focusing on work intensive thinking must only be done during working hours. So, practice removing your thinking cap after work. This hat can also be imagined by meditating, creating a thinking cap attitude prior to beginning work.

Also know that negativity is the mother of pessimism, and pessimism full blown is the invader of positive thinking, as well as the destroyer of good health. In order to turn this type of negative behavior around one must become an optimist whereby hope becomes a key player. To develop optimism it is important to consider everything as being beneficial to your wellbeing. In other words, instead of looking at a glass of water as being half empty, think of the same glass as being half full. This requires that one must find new hope - the kind of hope that is influenced by your change of attitude from negative thinking into positive thought patterns.

A good way to accomplish this is to find a special glass, fill it to the brim with water, and put it in a convenient spot where it can be seen every morning. Then, as you replenish the water that has evaporated think of it as replenishing your self-esteem, your hope. You can have fun finding ways of reciting positive affirmations while focusing on the glass filled with purple-colored water. Refilling the glass can become a ritual for developing self-esteem. It is important to realize that as the water evaporates, so too does your positive spirit diminish. Yes, it too, evaporates throughout the course of the day due to negativity presented throughout our ever-threatened universe.

Let your breathing assist you into hypnosis. Inhaling through the nose, think of your lungs filling up with purple oxygen. Then exhaling through the mouth, keep a relaxed rhythm going as you listen to these positive words. Let the realization of these images sink into your being while this vapor, this purple oxygen flows into your lungs, veins and throughout your nervous system. Remember that you are breathing to benefit your body, spirit and brain, as well as improving your character. Positively accept the fact that every lungful of oxygen is helping to enrich your spirit as well as your physiology, your entire personality. Feel and experience yourself becoming more confident - more and more filled with self-esteem. You can think of this as spiritual steam.   (continue)

Supernatural Power (continued)

Each time you inhale think of the oxygen as being a purple vapor coming into your spirit, cleansing you of all your impurities, of all your diseases. Now, imagine this purple vapor transforming into a purple aura surrounding your being. And now imagine this purple aura becoming a powerful enabling aura. Every time you breathe in, allow your purple aura to give off more positive energy, have it become more splendid. As you focus on visualizing your purple aura becoming more splendid, think of it as becoming your spiritual inner physician. It is now the most wonderful feeling you have felt in a long time.

In your subconscious, know that as these powerful words do their work, you will have become free from every emotional hurt, from all negative influences. You will sense the relief of every injury, of every negative influence that has had an effect on you. As you experience this special empowerment, know that you have become transformed for the better. As you continue to focus on your purple aura, know that you are protected from the influence of all harmful, or negative forces. In your subconscious, you know you are completely able to fulfill these objectives.

The true nature of your mind is that it wants to be healthy; it wants to be mentally sound. In that unique portion of your brain, there is a healing mechanism that is able to repair and regenerate itself. Your mind needs to feel successful; it strives to maintain a state of balance where every cell can function at its optimum performance. You know that your subconscious is able to do this, for it is the ultimate supernatural power. Deep down, you know that it knows what to do, and how to provide you with spiritual empowerment, naturally and instinctively. This is something that will stay with you even after you come out of this transforming, deep trance. Right now I'd like you to focus on trusting your empowerment. Feeling empowered, begin experiencing Unleashing Your Subconscious Power.

The solution, the magic key to accepting all this permanently, is to focus. Focus on the relaxed muscles, and the purple aura you are imagining now. Resolve right now to keep your muscles relaxed, rather than tense and restricted. Resolve in agreement with your subconscious mind to have all unnecessary tension become a thing of the past. Resolve to have your stress, your anxieties and all you unfounded fears become completely resolved. And now, even think about having these symptoms completely eradicated from your psyche, your behavior patterns. Imagine having all negativity dissipate allowing you to finally become sound-minded and focused as the complete person you know you can be. And now, in your own mind, truly accept the fact that your subconscious mind has agreed to handle this task. Actually, this is already acting to empower you now.   (continue)

Supernatural Power (continued)

Listen closely to these words as I say them to you: You feel peaceful; you feel very quiet emotionally. You feel calm physically, and you enjoy the peace, the quiet, and the secure feeling that permeates within your being. Accept this sense of security as becoming part of your personality. Your subconscious is registering all my words. The gentle words of my voice are being deeply engraved there as you listen intently to my suggestions. You are listening very intently as I proceed to empower your positive state of mind. While you concentrate on your purple aura, imagine that it is conducting a positive attitude. Imagine your inner physician as part of your colorful purple aura, protecting you. Have this new energy cover your entire body as you imagine it transforming into a dynamic, confidence-building, purple aura. This powerful, relaxing energy overwhelms you to the point you feel a tremendous confidence in yourself. Let yourself go. Let yourself feel whatever happens, because terrific things are taking place.

Still concentrating on your purple aura, you feel that your mind is free of all worry, free of problems and headaches. As you lie, free of tension, you rejoice in the sense of well being that this outer blue aura brings to you. Feel and experience this wonderful sensation, which spreads more and more throughout your body. You are lying comfortably with your eyes still closed; your arms and legs are flexible, relaxed. Now, concentrating on being loose and free imagine yourself as being completely surrounded with your purple aura. As you concentrate, imagine your purple aura as it begins to grow. Taking in deep breaths through your nose and exhaling through your mouth, let your entire body relax while lying in this comfortable position.

While you imagine your purple aura, concentrating as it continues to expand, you now envision yourself lying in the sand on a tropical beach. You can actually imagine yourself in a setting surrounded with palm trees. You are smiling as you see yourself basking in the sun, absorbing the warmth of the rays, the soothing rays of the afternoon sun. As you lie there, you imagine you are listening to the soothing, familiar sounds that a seashell might make, if you've ever placed one up to your ear and listened to the ocean's roar.

Still concentrating on this purple aura you are becoming more and more relaxed. More and more secure as you focus on the sounds of turbulent waves rolling in and out. Perhaps you may hear a seagull screeching, as it glides by overhead. You can even imagine a blue sky, with white, puffy clouds casting reflections on the calming ocean swells. Suddenly, you feel that your mind is free of all worry, free of daily problems and headaches.   (continue)

Supernatural Power (continued)

As you lie free of tension, you rejoice in the sense of well being that your blue aura brings you, which envelops you from head to foot. Feel and experience this wonderful warmth, this calming sensation as it spreads more and more throughout your body. Your subconscious has registered all my words. The gentle words of my voice have been deeply engraved there as you listen intently to my suggestions. You are listening very intently as I proceed to empower your positive state of mind.

Listen closely to these words as I say them to you: You feel protected, secure and full of high esteem as you accept this secure feeling that permeates within your being. Accept this sense of security as becoming part of your personality. As far as any problems with fear and anxiety are concerned, you are confident all is resolved. All episodes with panic, or unnecessary tension are finally over. Struggling with those uncomfortable feelings is a thing of the past. From now on you will be relieved of all tension caused by fear, pressure or stress, whether it be real or imagined.

You know you are capable of adjusting to this positive transformation, this new adjustment that is allowing you to become whole. You know deep down in your subconscious that you are able to cope with any situation. Yes, you are now able to cope with any uncomfortable situation that causes unnecessary tension because you know this power is within you. You know that this is inevitable because you have learned of nature's way of resolving your state of mind, your mental balance. When you come out of this very deep trance, there will be complete relaxation. You will experience complete relief from all unnecessary pain and anxiety. You will feel completely relaxed feeling relieved of any discomfort and stress, relieved of all unnecessary nervous tension, or pain.

In that safe place, deep within the darkest shadows of you mind, this supernatural empowerment process has taken place, even as I speak these positive words to you. Your entire nervous system is adjusting to my positive words, allowing your mind to become completely whole, completely balanced. Your subconscious acknowledges all this and readily accepts these adjustments. Yes, your subconscious mind is capable of making all the proper adjustments so that your body can become completely whole, completely balanced, completely empowered. Your entire nervous system is adjusting to my positive words, allowing your mind to become transformed to this state of positive empowerment. Your subconscious acknowledges all this and readily accepts these adjustments.

(continue)

Supernatural Power (continued)

Right now, I'd like you to visualize yourself as being completely empowered, completely transformed. Your mind is free of all worry, free of all stress, and daily problems. Feel and experience this wonderful sensation. Imagine this feeling as energy coming from your inner physician as it permeates throughout your body. Accept this inner physician, as it can actually perform cures and remedies that medical doctors sometimes cannot comprehend, or administer.
In your subconscious, know that as these positive words do their work, you will have become more and more relieved of every emotional hurt, of any mental disorders. You will sense the relief of every injury that has had a lasting effect on you. As you experience this special power, know that you have become positively transformed, permanently.

You are listening intently as I proceed, ultimately to program your mind to accept the fact that you are governed by a supernatural power. This power is so great, you can just imagine calling upon whatever you need and it will be provided for you. This all-empowering, positive mode you are now able to relate to, is called The Trance Zone. From now on, you will accept the fact that this remarkable, supernatural power is being bestowed upon you. To enforce your belief in this higher power, your subconscious mind acknowledges all this and will remember everything as a fact even after you come out of this empowering trance. Know that the beauty of inner growth is that is can be an endlessly enjoyable adventure. Remember that self-examination leads to self-insight. And self-insight leads to freedom of negative behavior patterns.

Your subconscious mind has recorded all of this information, and will acknowledge and process everything that has been said. As I slowly begin to count from 1 to 5, you will become better and better upon each count. 1 . . . You are feeling terrific knowing that you have finally been transformed. 2 . . . You remember everything that happened during this trance state. 3 . . . You feel happy that your life has changed for the better. 4 . . . You are totally relaxed, fully aware, and feeling empowered. 5 . . . You are awake and feeling ten times better than ever before. Finally, you are healthy, alert, and fully alive. It's time to open your eyes.

Note: *Both the "WORDS" of the SUBJECT and the "WORDS" of the HYPNOTHERAPIST are always shown in* **italics**. *The main difference between the dialog of the SUBJECT and the HYPNOTHERAPIST is that the subject's "WORDS" are always shown in the "first person."*

APPLICATION OF ACTUAL SCRIPTS (continued)

EXAMPLE 1: To have the subject *"Come Out"*

The way you are feeling refreshed now is the way you can always expect to feel. Your subconscious mind has recorded this and will remember everything that has been said. When I count to five, you will open your eyes feeling alert, refreshed and alive. 1 . . . 2 . . . every part of you is better than ever before, 3 . . . you are feeling alert and refreshed, 4 . . . you are alert, refreshed and fully alive, 5 . . . Open your eyes.

EXAMPLE 2: To have the subject *"Come Out"*

In that safe place, deep within the darkest shadows of you mind, this supernatural process has already taken place. As I slowly begin to count from one to five, you will become better and better upon each count. 1 . . . You are feeling terrific knowing that you have finally been transformed. 2 . . . You remember everything that happened during this trance state. 3 . . . You feel happy having your positive personality. 4 . . . You are totally relaxed, fully aware, and feeling empowered. 5 . . . You are awake and feeling ten times better than ever before. Finally, you are healthy, alert, and fully alive. It's time to open your eyes.

EXAMPLE 3: To have the subject *"Come Out"*

You are feeling fabulously well experiencing high self-esteem. Your subconscious mind has recorded this and will remember everything that has been said. When you hear me say: it's time to open your eyes you will awaken, feeling happy and filled with your spiritual steam. It's time to open your eyes.

As a hypnotherapist it would be good experience to practice writing, reciting and recording your own scripts. It may seem difficult at first, but with commitment and practice, it will be possible to adlib an entire half hour script – making up the words to suit the particular patient's disorder.

(Review PSYCHOLOGICAL TOOLS in Chapter Three.)

PART FOUR

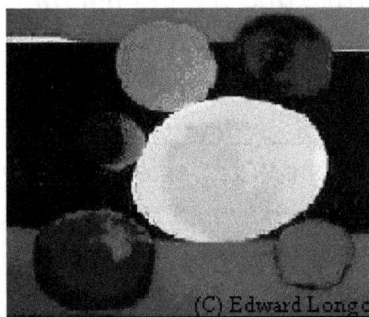

(C) Edward Longo

CHAPTER SEVEN
7

HYPNOTHERAPY
INDUCTION
TECHNIQUES

---

7   INDUCTION TECHNIQUES
AS HYPNOTHERAPIST:

By utilizing the applications, practicing the inductions, and incorporating various techniques the hypnotherapist is then able to "Go Into" <u>The Trance Zone</u> and gain access to subconscious programming. The secret to tapping the depths of the mind is to go into the subconscious, where the true source of power rules.

This is where you can unleash the power of your subconscious mind, and change negative habits of thought and action into what you desire them to be. This is how you can alter programming for the better; this is how you prepare yourself, or your patient's through the use of "Psychological Tools."

. . . EJL

CHAPTER SEVEN

7

HYPNOTHERAPY INDUCTION TECHNIQUES
Example Inductions

INDUCTION TECHNIQUES
As Hypnotherapist

Due to the affects parents have on us in early childhood, the influences of society, and negativity from friends and associates, we often become undermined with suggestions of incompetence and failure. Subconsciously, that subliminal tape recording of years past kicks in and plays the derogatory messages over and over, sabotaging our mind.   Consequently, that negative influence becomes the underlying part of us that criticizes, edits, and judges everything, thereby limiting our capabilities. (More information about Hypnotherapy Induction Techniques my be found in The Trance Zone Hypnosis Manual.)

It is through the subconscious mind that we can gain the key to insight, self-esteem and success. The subconscious is the intrinsic substance of the mind – it is the mother lode, the more powerful part of us, that stronger part of our individuality that is really the dominant force.

Through the practice of hypnotherapy we are able to gain access to knowledge and human understanding, the likes of which millions of people, including most doctors and psychologists, may never acquire. Ultimately, through the application of hypnotherapy and hypnosis, there is no limit to what we can achieve. It may even become possible to become a virtual genius, provided enough time was spent in effort, perseverance, and total commitment.

(continue)

<u>INDUCTION TECHNIQUES</u> (continued)

The use of hypnotherapy is not some form of hocus-pocus. It is one of the most powerful, effective ways to gain access to that supreme part of you that, probably, has never been programmed properly. Hypnosis has been used by psychiatrists during World War II to treat wounded soldiers, and was used additionally to banish the combat traumas that caused hysterical paralysis, as well as amnesia. Ever since 1958, when the American Medical Association approved the use of hypnosis, it has been used successfully to treat phobias, addiction, insomnia, pain, depression, PTSD, and neurological problems.

Hypnotherapy is still being widely practiced by psychiatrists, surgeons, doctors, and hypnotherapists alike, to treat disease - and because its effect is organic, hypnosis is truly a marvel of mind over mind. When used properly, it can be used as a tool to investigate past lives, probe into the problems of the psyche, and even traverse and envision what the future may have in store. The practice of hypnotherapy is not a mere mental procedure. Hypnosis has turned out to become a supernatural phenomenon that continues to behoove the average person, even to this day. Becoming hypnotized to overcome issues is definitely the wave of the future, where more and more people want to grow intellectually - psychologically, as well as physiologically. Finally, health, wealth, and the pursuit of happiness can be achieved by all who dare to become involved in one of the most revolutionary forms of treatment of the 21st century.

Here, the Induction Techniques may vary, depending on the subject's needs, and how you, as hypnotherapist decide to treat the problem. Some hypnotherapist's use a spinning wheel, or a pendulum, while some use flickering lights; still, a few employ the snap of a finger to induce posthypnotic suggestions, while others use a certain touch. All of these techniques are acceptable and okay to use. However, I have found the techniques listed below to be highly effective, while they quickly find a direct path to the subconscious.

With permission, the hypnotherapist's inductions may be recorded for the subject's, or patient's use for listening at home. If practicing self-hypnosis, there is nothing to memorize. Simply tape your preferred inductions (best recorded the "first person,") and listen to them repeatedly, preferably with headphones.

<u>INDUCTION TECHNIQUES</u> (continued)

<u>Posthypnotic Suggestions</u> are the "CUES," messages, key words, or triggers induced by the hypnotist to the subject in the hypnotic state. The purpose of the hypnotist's suggestions is to have them carry over, thus influencing the subject in the awakened state – they are also used as a trigger to aid the subject in returning to the hypnotic state. For example, the hypnotist can give the subject a word, such as "<u>golden nugget</u>" under hypnosis, and upon being given that command in the awakened state, the subject will return to the preceding hypnotic trance state. Similarly, snapping the fingers three times, while the subject repeats, "<u>I can do</u>" three times under hypnosis, can induce self-confidence when the command is executed in the awakened state.

<u>Posthypnotic Suggestions</u> act as tools, in order to enable progressive treatment. In this instance, forming *"the hypnotic eye"* would enable the subject to rapidly "Go Into" *<u>The Trance Zone</u>* in subsequent sessions. Invariably, the subject's eyes will close very rapidly, inducing the trance.

Since all posthypnotic suggestions become effective when induced during the trance state, have the subject *"Go into" <u>The Trance Zone</u>*, and repeatedly give the subject the key words: *This is how you "Go Into" <u>The Trance Zone</u>*. After a few visits, the subject will easily go into hypnosis.

<u>WRITING CUSTOM SCRIPTS</u>

<u>As Hypnotherapist</u>

As a hypnotherapist, practice memorizing and performing the inductions below on your subjects. Imagine seeing the results of each patient becoming healthy, or fulfilling their dreams, their hearts desires. Although it is best to perform the inductions from memory they are so complex it would be quite difficult. Select your favorite script, and practice memorizing it until you are ready for another. However, don't rely too heavily on memorization. Something to consider is that, since the subject's eyes will be closed, you could actually read the inductions from printed pages, or cards.

Note: In becoming a professional hypnotherapist, it would be good experience to practice writing, reciting and recording your own trance scripts. It may seem difficult at first, but with commitment and practice, it will be possible to adlib an entire half hour script – making up the words to suit the particular patient's disorder. Listed below are examples of a variety of hypnotic scripts.

WRITING CUSTOM SCRIPTS (continued)

Typical Induction Technique (with the subject sitting or lying)
First, have the subject *"Go Into" The Trance Zone* as follows:

Instruct the subject to encircle the thumb and forefinger to form *"the hypnotic eye."* Then have the subject place the *"eyes up to the eyebrows,"* close them, and give *"deep yawn."* Then give the posthypnotic suggestion, which automatically becomes a "CUE", subconsciously, to go into the trance state.

EXAMPLE:
HYPNOTHERAPIST:

This is how you "Go Into" The Trance Zone. Every time I give you this message, it will be easier for you to go into hypnosis. Concentrating while forming "the hypnotic eye," "Go Into" The Trance Zone, and then go deeper and deeper into hypnosis.

Behavior Modification Technique (with subject sitting or lying)
First, have the subject *"Go Into" The Trance Zone* as follows:
HYPNOTHERAPIST:

I'd like you to lift your "eyes up to the eyebrows," and when you feel like it, close them. Give a "deep yawn," and form "the hypnotic eye" by placing my thumb and forefinger together. Now repeat this after me: "This is how I "Go Into" The Trance Zone." Very good – that is how you "Go Into" The Trance Zone, where only good things happen. In that wide opening to your subconscious, you are listening intently to my voice.

Your arms and legs are flexible, relaxed. As I count down from 30 by 2's, continue breathing evenly, inhaling through your nose and exhaling through your mouth. 30, 28, 26, 24 . . . With each breath you sink deeper and deeper and deeper into a relaxed state of mind. 22, 20, 18, 16 . . . You no longer want anything. Become passive as you listen to my voice. Let yourself go . . . 14 . . . 12 . . . 10 . . . 8 . . . 6 . . . 4 . . . 2 . . . Zero.

Nothing bothers or distracts you. Nothing bad or unusual is going to happen. Your head is clear. Your mind is free of all problems. You rejoice in this sense of peace and wellbeing that envelops you from head to foot. Feel this wonderful relaxation which spreads more and more throughout your body. Feel the new looseness and weightlessness of your body. In this wonderful state of peace, you have an opening to the subconscious -- wider and wider this opening is becoming. Your subconscious is registering all my words. The gentle words of my voice are being deeply engraved there as you listen intently to my suggestions.

Behavior Modification Technique (continued)

In that wide opening to your subconscious mind, you will remember how great it feels when your imagination takes over, how it can make you feel better about yourself. When you come out of this, you will remember everything and make use of it in every aspect of your life.

As you are resting comfortably, you will notice that your eyes are closed tight, very tight. They are stuck so tight you are not able to open them. In a moment I will ask you to try to open them - you will not be able to do so. You will find they are sealed tight; they are stuck firmly together. You may be able to manage the muscle groups around your eyes, but not your eyelids. No matter how hard you try, you will be unable to open your eyes.

When I count down from 3 to zero, you will find it impossible to open your eyes and you will go deeper into hypnosis. 3 . . . Your eyelids are sealed tight, 2 . . . They are stuck tight, 1 . . . They are stuck firmly together, Zero . . . Try, but you are unable to open them. Stop trying, and go deeper into hypnosis.

Spinning Crystal Technique (with the subject sitting or lying)

First, have the subject *"Go Into"* <u>*The Trance Zone*</u> and proceed as follows:

Instruct the subject to focus on a spinning multifaceted crystal as you suspended it on a string, above the subject's eyes. Then, instruct the subject to keep staring at the object, lift the *"eyes up to the eyebrows,"* then close them, and give *"deep yawn."*

Next recite: *This is how you "Go Into"* <u>*The Trance Zone.*</u>

Then, have the subject *"inhale through the nose,"* and exhale counting down from 30 by 2's, relaxing the body more and more, until reaching zero.

As an alternate method to the Spinning Crystal, the hypnotherapist may place a multifaceted crystal within the fingers forming *"the hypnotic eye"* and slowly raise it up and above the subject's head, and quickly lowering it down. Most often, this will trigger the eyes to close, creating a trance.

Review the following techniques and practice reading them aloud before initiating them. It is important that your voice flows rhythmically when performing all hypnotic inductions. In practicing the examples as demonstrated below, you will eventually be able to develop your own personalized inductions. Whenever ending a hypnotic trance it is advisable to use one of the various *"Come Out"* procedures after every hypnosis session.

WRITING CUSTOM SCRIPTS (continued)

EXAMPLE INDUCTION – #1:
HYPNOTHERAPIST
Have the subject *"Go Into"* The Trance Zone as above then recite:

This radiant, pure light within you is energizing and transforming your whole being in such positive ways multitudes of miracles are taking place mentally, physically and emotionally. This inner, illuminated light has created within you a sound mind and body, and is curing you of all disease and disorders. As you concentrate on feeling the warmth of my hands, think only of tranquility as you continue to breathe deeply, steadily, and evenly. As you listen to my voice, you are confident, having the knowledge that you are in good hands – hands that have very effective healing powers. Know that I am here to activate, stimulate and rejuvenate all the elements of you mind, body and spirit. Concentrate on this knowledge as you breathe deeply, having the incoming oxygen replenish your entire immune system, your entire spiritual being. Know that my energy is flowing through me to you, in order that you may become well. Know this, believe it, and accept it as a gift to you coming from the radiant light from above.

EXAMPLE INDUCTION – #2:
HYPNOTHERAPIST
Have the subject *"Go Into"* The Trance Zone as above then recite:

As you continue breathing deeply and calmly, you know in your heart that your ideal state of mind is that of calmness and tranquility. In this peaceful state that encompasses your whole being, you feel almost as if time has stopped for you. All worries are put aside, all tension and pain has left your body. In that wide opening to your subconscious, you feel you are in complete control of the healing powers of your own immune system, as well as all your vital organs. In this state of tranquility, your subconscious mind prevents any disease from disrupting your mental or physical health.

EXAMPLE INDUCTION – #3:
HYPNOTHERAPIST
Have the subject *"Go Into"* The Trance Zone as above then recite:

Through the powers of this radiant, illuminating light flowing through me, I command your subconscious to become free of smoking and all the undesirable habits that go with it. I command my subconscious mind to free you of being possessed by this disgusting and depressing need to smoke. By the power of this illuminating light flowing through me, I now release all the bondage, addictions, and cravings that once held you hostage.

WRITING CUSTOM SCRIPTS (continued)

The hypnosis trance script below is an example of how an induction trance script for insomnia may be written. (Delivery time: ten to fifteen minutes.)

Overcoming Insomnia / Inducing peaceful sleep

Have the subject "*Go Into*" <u>*The Trance Zone*</u> as follows:

HYPNOTHERAPIST

I'd like you to form "the hypnotic eye" by placing the thumb and forefinger of either hand together, and place your hand at your side. This is the eye to your subconscious, which puts you into The Trance Zone. Now, I'd like you to lift your "eyes up to the eyebrows" and, when you feel like it, let your eyelids close. Keeping your eyes up take in a " deep yawn" and recite: "This is how I go into The Trance Zone."

Very good -- that is how you "Go Into" The Trance Zone, where only good things happen. In that wide opening to your subconscious, you are listening intently to my voice. Your arms and legs are flexible, relaxed. Please note that it is important to focus on the hypnotic eye with the three fingers extended. Use of the hypnotic eye will be helpful in having it serve as a tool. With practice this will become your source of personal self-esteem, your positive secret weapon.

Your arms and legs are flexible, relaxed. As we both count down from 12 by 2's, continue breathing evenly, inhaling through your nose and exhaling through your mouth. When I say the number 12, take in a deep breath and begin counting down aloud. 12, 10, 8 . . . With each breath you sink deeper into a relaxed state of mind. 6, 4 . . . the lower the number the deeper you go into hypnosis. 2 . . . Zero.

The deeper you go into hypnosis you go deeper into hypnosis. As you continue to listen to my voice just allow yourself to become open minded and completely open to my directions, positive suggestions, and guided imagery. Soon, these words will open your doorway to becoming transformed in an extremely powerful way. It is very important to note that rhythmic breathing is also used as a tool for going deeper into hypnosis. The calmer the rhythm established during this hypnosis session, the deeper the hypnotic state will become.

So, in addition to focusing on the hypnotic eye, please focus on deep, relaxed breathing throughout this session. Know that you are connected to the source that will provide you with all the security, self-confidence, and emotional assuredness you will ever need to make positive changes permanently. Right now hardly anything distracts you.

(continue)

Overcoming Insomnia (continued)

Hardly anything will interfere with you going deeper into hypnosis. Only positive changes are going to take place. Only good things are going to happen as your mind becomes clear. Your mind is free of all tension, free of all problems. You welcome this sense of freedom and well being that relieves stress from head to foot. Feel this wonderful relaxation as you experience the looseness and weightlessness of your body; sinking deeper, and deeper. Now let your fingers loosen.

Imagine every part of your body becoming so relaxed it seems like jelly. Allow this relaxation to balance your entire nervous system, your complete immune system, as you focus on allowing your mind to come to complete rest. You are free of all worry, free of all tension as you drift off into your hypnotic trance. Deeper and deeper you go into this deep trance state; deeper and deeper you go into hypnosis. The deeper you go into hypnosis, the deeper you go into this trance state. Deeper and deeper, you drift off into your beautiful, restful hypnotic trance.

My words have an especially powerful influence on the neuro-psychological system within you. The beautiful words and special tones of my voice have been orchestrated to help stimulate your body's entire healing mechanism. These special words act as a powerful medicine to your complete mental system. These hypnotic words are being registered in your subconscious, right down to the complex activity of your nerves. These hypnotic sounds of my voice are actually performing healing, harmony and coordination within your entire body. Your entire nervous system is adjusting to my positive words, allowing your mind to become at ease.

Let your breathing assist you into hypnosis. Each time you inhale imagine receiving renewed vitality from the source of life that surrounds us – the universal energy which nourishes the plants and trees, which holds the birds in flight, and which blows the winds from the four corners of the earth. Each time you exhale remind yourself that you are also emptying away all disease, nervous disorders and feelings of negativity. Continue feeling relaxed as you experience letting go of all tight muscles, all unwelcome stress.

Let the realization of these images sink into your being while focusing on your breathing. Reassure yourself that you are not only breathing to retain life, you are breathing to live life, and to live life more abundantly. Remember that you are breathing to benefit your body, spirit and brain, as well as improving your character. Positively accept the fact that every lungful of oxygen is helping to enrich your spirit as well as your physiology, your entire personality. Feel and experience yourself becoming more confident, more filled with self-esteem. You can think of this as spiritual steam.   (continue)

<u>Overcoming Insomnia</u> (continued)

In your subconscious, you know you are completely able to fulfill these objectives. The true nature of your mind is that it wants to be healthy; it wants to be mentally sound. In that unique portion of your brain, there is a healing mechanism that is able to repair and regenerate itself. Your mind needs to feel successful; it strives to maintain a state of balance where every cell can function at its optimum performance. You know that your subconscious is able to do this, for it is the ultimate supernatural power. Deep down, you know that it knows what to do, and how to provide you with spiritual empowerment, instinctively. This is something that will stay with you even after you come out of this deep trance.

Right now I'd like you to focus on trusting your relaxed state. The solution, the magic key to accepting all this permanently, is to focus. Focus on the relaxed muscles, and the purple aura you are imagining now. Resolve right now to keep your muscles relaxed, rather than tense and restricted. Resolve in agreement with your subconscious mind to have all unnecessary tension become a thing of the past. Resolve to have your stress, your anxieties and all you unfounded fears become completely resolved. Imagine having all negativity dissipate allowing you to finally become free from bondage. And now, in your own mind, truly accept the fact that your subconscious mind has agreed to handle this task. Have this renewed energy cover your entire body as you imagine it transforming into a dynamic, confidence-building, purple aura. This powerful, relaxing energy overwhelms you to the point you feel a tremendous confidence in yourself.

Right now, I'd like you to visualize yourself as being magnificently transformed. Your mind is free of all worry, free of all stress, and daily problems. Feel and experience this wonderful sensation. Imagine your inner physician as being part of your healing process, protecting you. Imagine this healing as energy coming from your inner physician as it permeates throughout your body.

You know you are capable of adjusting to this positive transformation, this new adjustment that is allowing you to become whole. You know deep down in your subconscious that you are able to cope with any situation. Yes, you are now able to cope with any uncomfortable situation that causes unnecessary tension because you know this power is within you. When you come out of this very deep trance you will experience complete relief from all unnecessary pain and anxiety. You will feel completely relaxed and free of any discomfort and stress, relieved of all unnecessary nervous tension, or pain. In your subconscious, know that you have become more and more relieved of every emotional hurt, of any mental disorders.

(continue)

Overcoming Insomnia (continued)

This all-empowering, positive mode you are now able to relate to, is called The Trance Zone. Your subconscious has adjusted to my positive words, and will acknowledge and process everything that has been said. From now on, you will accept the fact that this remarkable, supernatural power is being bestowed upon you. To enforce your belief in this higher power, your subconscious has acknowledged all this and will remember everything as a fact. Know that the beauty of inner growth is that it can be an endlessly enjoyable adventure. Remember that self-examination leads to self-insight. And self-insight leads to freedom of negative behavior patterns.

Even after you come out of this deep trance you will remember that forming "the hypnotic eye" is the key to unleashing the power of your subconscious mind. Whenever you call upon this image hidden knowledge is brought to light. As you look deeper and deeper within your spirit, you draw wisdom from the depths of your subconscious mind. All knowledge is there for you. All channels of guidance are opened to you, especially spiritual guidance. Everything you want to know is revealed. Everything is made clear; everything is exposed.

As far as any problems with sleeping are concerned, you are confident all is resolved. Any bouts with insomnia are finally over. Struggling in order to find peaceful sleep is a thing of the past. Now, whenever you lay down for the night, you realize that sleeping is the way your body recuperates. You also know that sleep is inevitable because it is nature's way of replenishing your strength and your state of mental balance. Whenever you decide to fall asleep your sleep is deep and unencumbered. Whenever you awaken, there is complete rest and complete relief from all kinds of stress. Focusing on this subconscious state you envision yourself as the person you have always dreamed you could be. Your subconscious mind has already allowed you to feel better about yourself. When you awaken, you will remember everything that happened during this trance.

In that safe place, deep within the darkest shadows of you mind, this supernatural process has already taken place. As I slowly begin to count from one to five, you will become better and better upon each count. 1 . . . You are feeling terrific knowing that you have finally been transformed. 2 . . . You remember everything that happened during this trance state. 3 . . . You feel happy having your positive personality. 4 . . . You are totally relaxed, fully aware, and feeling empowered. 5 . . . You are awake and feeling ten times better than ever before. Finally, you are healthy, alert, and fully alive. It's time to open your eyes.

CUSTOM TRANCE SCRIPT

Lose Weight Permanently – A Customized Trance Script
Fulfilling The Subject's Needs For A Trim Waist

Have the patient "*Go Into*" *The Trance Zone* as follows:
HYPNOTHERAPIST

I'd like you to form "the hypnotic eye" by placing the thumb and forefinger of either hand together, and place your hand at your side. This is the eye to your subconscious, which puts you into The Trance Zone. Now, I'd like you to lift your "eyes up to the eyebrows" and, when you feel like it, let your eyelids close. Keeping your eyes up take in a "deep yawn" and recite: "This is how I go into The Trance Zone."

Very good -- that is how you "Go Into" The Trance Zone, where only good things happen. In that wide opening to your subconscious, you are listening intently to my voice. Your arms and legs are flexible, relaxed. Please note that it is important to focus on the hypnotic eye with the three fingers extended. Use of the hypnotic eye will be helpful in having it serve as a tool. With practice this will become your source of personal self-esteem, your positive secret weapon.

As I count down from 30 by 2's, continue breathing evenly, inhaling through your nose and exhaling through your mouth. 30, 28, 26, 24 . . . With each breath you sink deeper and deeper and deeper into a relaxed state of mind. 22, 20, 18, 16 . . . You no longer want anything. Become passive as you listen to my voice. Let yourself go . . . 14 . . . 12 . . . 10 . . . 8 . . . 6 . . . 4 . . . 2 . . . Zero.

Let it be . . . Let it happen. Nothing bothers or distracts you. Nothing bad or unusual is going to happen. Your head is clear. Your mind is free of all problems. You rejoice in this sense of peace and well being that envelops you from head to foot. Feel this wonderful relaxation which spreads more and more throughout your body. Feel the new looseness and weightlessness of your body.

In this wonderful state of peace, you have an opening to the subconscious -- wider and wider this opening is becoming. Your subconscious is registering all my words. The gentle words of my voice are being deeply engraved there as you listen intently to my suggestions.

You are listening very intently as I proceed with care. Listen closely to these words as I say them to you: You feel peaceful; you feel very quiet emotionally. You feel calm physically, and you enjoy the peace, the quiet, and the calm that exudes from within you.

(continue)

Lose Weight Permanently (continued)

In that wide opening to your subconscious, you are listening intently to my voice. Perhaps you already know about your subconscious mind's extraordinary powers of self-healing, and how the right side of your brain controls the functioning of your entire body. The right side of your brain, the subconscious mind, knows how to regulate your breathing even while you are sleeping, and knows how to regulate your circulatory system, how to carry the right nutrients to all the parts of your body that need them. This brilliant part of your mind also knows how to instruct every cell in your body to heal itself, to improve, to feel more comfortable and to be healthy and sound, cell by magnificent cell. And I know that your body is healing itself now, as your mind knows just how to accelerate the healing that is taking place, balancing your normal body weight.

Still listening to my voice, your entire body has become more relaxed, feeling free and secure. While your muscles become free of tension, my voice is going deeper into that opening to you subconscious. Now that you are totally relaxed and feeling completely free of tension, imagine all your guilt, worries, frustrations, and hostilities leaving your body, permanently.

Imagine that all that negativity is flowing out of your lungs and pores like poisonous gases leaving you feeling completely refreshed, recharged, and rejuvenated. Right now, know in your mind that you fully and freely release all grudges held from the past. Fully and freely loosen and let go of all anger, resentment and pent-up emotional disorders. Feel the relief of unloading all this excess baggage from your mind. From this day forward your load is finally light. Your burdens are light and all your worries and problems have just become trivial.

You may remember back to a time in your life that you became ill and had to go to a doctor to be treated. But your subconscious mind knows that it was not the doctor, or the medicine that healed you – it was you and your body that ultimately healed you, cell by incredible cell. Yes, your subconscious has the intelligence and the power to heal anything inside of you on an intercellular basis – even when it comes to losing those extra pounds.

You may have read or heard, or perhaps you know from your own experience that athletes need to take great care in order for their bodies to grow strong, and to recuperate when overworked. And as you rest your body now, like an athlete rests, your body can become stronger and healthier, revitalizing your nerves, your blood, and even your brain cells. And although your physical body is always being affected by gravity, it doesn't have to follow that you have to gain excessive weight.

(continue)

Lose Weight Permanently (continued)

And I don't know if you have already felt certain sensations in your body, signaling that the healing process has already started, but you can be sure that while you are in this deep, resting trance state, your body is already healing itself. You can enjoy feeling relaxed, knowing your body can accelerate and improve your immune system even now, as you enjoy this rest. Know for sure that you can rely on your inner self; that you can count on that part of you in your subconscious that knows exactly what to do, and exactly how to do it.

Perhaps you remember a time when you had a bout with the flu. You probably went to a doctor for treatment, but then even as you slept and played and worked, your body did all the healing. While your body has a tremendous ability to heal itself, the subconscious mind actually serves as the regulator of every possible part, every possible function. Not only does your subconscious have the ability to perform all the healing you need, it has the capability to initiate peaceful rest and sleep when called upon.

Your subconscious mind is capable of extraordinary recouping powers, and endless capacities, even while you enjoy your peaceful trance. You <u>know</u> that, and you can continue to allow your body to rejuvenate while you relax and enjoy feeling peaceful. That deep place in your subconscious mind acknowledges all this and remembers to call upon this information. And even after you come out of this exhilarating trance state, you can trust your ability to initiate healing whenever it is needed. When you go to bed at night, you take delight in the fact that sleeping serves to replenish your entire body, hour after hour, cell by remarkable cell.

You are listening intently as I proceed, ultimately to program your mind to accept a positive attitude toward your weight. The positive mode you are now able to relate to is called The Trance Zone. From now on, when I mention the word <u>waist</u> you will immediately <u>think</u> of having a trim <u>waist</u>. Even though there has been a lull in your activity within the past few years, the fact remains that you are still that physically fit person you always knew could identify with, even during the lulls in your activity. The fact that your activity in sports has subsided only means you have had less time for it. Since your life has been so demanding, and stress-full, it has begun to diminish the drive you had for keeping in shape.

But your drive has always been there. And it is this distinguishable drive of yours that is going to get you back on track. Now it is time to focus your energy and muster up enough drive to get you to get into tip-top shape. From now on, you will allow yourself the luxury of being trim and fit, even if it only means exercising moderately, or cutting back on the many harmful foods.   (continue)

<u>Lose Weight Permanently</u> (continued)

Specifically, diminishing the weight you have gained at your <u>waist</u> is something you already know is being resolved. You know you have been putting this off for too long, and, subconsciously, you know you are in the process of losing those unnecessary pounds around your <u>waist</u>, as well as other parts of your physique that may have become too excessive. To enforce your belief of knowing you will always keep your <u>waist</u> thin, you acknowledge, even just thinking about it, that your <u>waist</u> is adjusting and becoming trim and ideally thin. In fact, even as you listen to my voice, you can feel your <u>waist</u> muscles tugging, and tightening, indicating that they are responding my suggestions, as well as to your desire to become thin. You agree that you have the ability to keep your <u>waist</u> thin and trim. When it comes to being physically fit, you are not the type to let yourself go.

You are always giving yourself a nudge, a push, or facing one more challenge to enable yourself to remain physically fit. You feel that it is right for you to maintain being physically fit, even if it is only to please yourself. But you go beyond that. In your subconscious mind, you know you are not happy with less than one hundred percent enthusiasm, physically and emotionally. In keeping with your ideals, when it comes to being in top condition, you always could find a way of maintaining your best form exhibiting personal appeal, especially when it comes to influencing and impressing those around you.

The true nature of your mind is that it wants to be sound; it wants to be healthy. In that unique portion of your brain, there is a healing system that is able to repair and regenerate itself. Your mind needs to be healthy; it strives to maintain a state of balance where every cell can function at its optimum performance. Your conscious thoughts have little to do with maintaining this mental process. Actually, your conscious thinking process is more likely to hinder your natural ability to heal, than it would be able to escalate your health and well being. The magic key, the solution to having a fit body and a sound mind, is to get your conscious thoughts out of the way. Know that your subconscious knows what you need, and that it knows how and when to do it, naturally, instinctively.

The sound of my voice has an especially powerful influence on your neuro-psychological system. The beautiful rhythm, smooth tones, and softness of my voice have been executed deliberately to help stimulate your body's entire healing mechanism. These innovative sounds of my voice act as a powerful medicine to your complete mental system, right down to the complex activity of your nerves.

(continue)

Lose Weight Permanently (continued)

The true nature of your mind is that it wants to be sound; it wants to be healthy. In that unique portion of your brain, there is a healing system that is able to repair and regenerate itself. Your mind needs to be healthy; it strives to maintain a state of balance where every cell can function at its optimum performance. Your conscious thoughts have little to do with maintaining this mental process. Actually, your conscious thinking process is more likely to hinder your natural ability to heal, than it would be able to escalate your health and well being. The magic key, the solution to having a fit body and a sound mind, is to get your conscious thoughts out of the way, so that your subconscious can do what it knows how to do, and when to do it, naturally, instinctively.

In that safe place, deep within the darkest shadows of you mind, this supernatural healing process is taking place, even as I speak these health-rendering words to you. Right now, I'd like you to visualize yourself as being completely well. In your subconscious, know that as these sounds do their work, you will have become more and more healed of every emotional hurt, all mental illness, and every injury that has had a lasting effect on you. As you experience this special healing know that your physique has become more fit. Know that, even as we progress, your <u>waist</u> is becoming thinner, and will become more, and more trim, as time passes.

Imagine a large softgel containing a liquid tranquilizer being lodged in the upper portion of your brain. Let it become loose and slowly travel down the head, and settle into the back of your neck. Now, let the softgel dissolve, allowing the liquid tranquilizer to flow down your throat and settle there. Feel the liquid dissolving into your throat. And now, allow the liquid tranquilizer to settle into every part of your body starting from your throat, and seeping down to the bottom of your feet. Feel its tranquilizing effect as it seeps down your chest and arms. Feel its loosening and healing effects as it seeps into every muscle, every ligament and into every joint.

Now, breathing in deeply, take in full breaths as if you can picture the oxygen filling your lungs. As you continue to breathe deeply, imagine the oxygen as a magic healing vapor. The deeper you breathe, the deeper this healing vapor circulates into your entire body. The more oxygen you take in, the more you feel the effect of its healing powers. Visualize a clear picture of this healing vapor going into your lungs and circulating throughout your nervous system.

(continue)

Lose Weight Permanently (continued)

Imagine every part of your body becoming so relaxed it seems like jelly. Allow this liquid tranquilizer to relieve every pain, every arthritic condition, every restrictive feeling in your body. Allow this tranquilizer to balance your entire nervous system, your complete immune system, as you focus on allowing your mind to come to complete rest. You are free of all worry, free of all tension as you drift off into your hypnotic trance. Deeper and deeper you go into this deep trance state; deeper and deeper you go into hypnosis. The deeper you go into hypnosis, the deeper you go into this trance state. Deeper and deeper, you drift off into your beautiful, restful hypnotic trance.

To enforce your belief in knowing you will always keep your waist thin, you acknowledge that your waist has adjusted to becoming thin. In fact, even as you listen to my voice, you can feel your waist muscles tugging, and tightening, indicating that they are responding my suggestions, as well as to your desire to become thin. You acknowledge that you have the ability to keep your waist thin. When it comes to being physically fit, you are not the type to let yourself go.

In your subconscious you know you are completely able to perform, to fulfill your ideals, when it comes to being in condition and keeping your waist trim. Know in your heart, and accept it in your mind, that you are a physically fit, attractive human being. Your subconscious mind has recorded all this and will remember everything that has been said.

The way you are feeling secure and refreshed right now is the way you can always expect to feel. Your subconscious mind has recorded this and will remember everything that has been said. In that safe place, deep within the darkest shadows of you mind, this supernatural process has already taken place. When I count to five, you will open your eyes feeling alert, refreshed and alive. 1 . . . 2 . . . every part of you is better than ever before, 3 . . . you are feeling alert and refreshed, 4 . . . you are alert, refreshed and fully alive, 5 . . . Open your eyes.

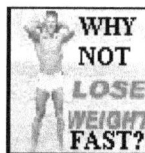

Why Not Lose Weight Fast?

CHAPTER EIGHT
8

POSITIVE SUGGESTIONS
& MIND-ALTERING
AFFIRMATIONS

---

8   MIND-ALTERING
AFFIRMATIONS:

The first thing I explained to a new patient Paul X during his initial visit was that in order to enter the trance state of hypnosis patients do not "go under" hypnosis. That is, he, as the subject would "Go Iinto" the hypnotic trance, rather than to going under my spell. Being overcome by the hypnotist's spell, I explained, was a definitive misconception of how hypnosis was performed.

In actuality, the healing power that hypnotherapy provides is directly incumbent upon the spiritual harmony that you, as Hypnotherapist, uncover in tandem with the patient.

Mission Statement:
Inspire The Injured Spirit And You Can Dissipate Any Disorder, Even Disease. . . .
. . EJL

CHAPTER EIGHT
8

POSITIVE SUGGESTIONS &
MIND-ALTERING AFFIRMATIONS

INDUCING POSITIVE SUGGESTIONS &
MIND-ALTERING AFFIRMATIONS

Find the positive force that overcomes the conflicting, negative weakness, and you have discovered the key to positive transformation.

Self-Hypnosis and Behavior Modification

Infiltrating the subconscious mind by bombarding it with new truths enables us the power to change for the betterment of our lives. Words are especially powerful when spoken audibly. They can instill belief or discredit belief, creating positive or negative energy. The most effective way to instill belief is to bypass the conscious mind, which criticizes, and deliver messages into the subconscious, where they become accepted without reasoning.

Through the practice of hypnosis, it is feasible to break a bad habit, which is a negative, degenerative habit, by replacing it with a good habit – which becomes a beneficial, positive habit. Everyone develops habits, but some are positive, while others are negative. The problems rise when our negative habits control us - for they begin inducing demoralizing, and abusive, self-defeating traits. They are called "bad habits" because they are bad for us, personally, and sometimes just as bad for those around us. Whether falling into patterns of negative conditioning, or self-destruction – reprogramming our thoughts can be successfully used to alter the defeatist personality. Through the practice of Mind-Altering Suggestions, persons can actually become enabled to alter their personality traits.

(continue)

POSITIVE SUGGESTIONS & AFFIRMATIONS (continued)
Mind-altering Suggestions and Affirmations

The only truth the conscious mind knows is what it has received from its subconscious, whether they are lies, or not. Since everything delivered into the subconscious is not always recognized as the truth many persons go around acknowledging distorted truths within their established belief system. Sometimes it is those lies that sabotage the mind, causing various diseases and disorders. This is why hypnotherapy is so valuable – the professional hypnotherapist is capable of replacing the lies that have often infiltrated the mind, and belief system. By implanting suggestions containing the actual truth the hypnotherapist becomes a sort of alchemist. Hence, truthful, positive messages are delivered, subconsciously, and transformation is soon accomplished . . . EJL

Too Many People Are Skeptical About Hypnosis

The first thing I explained to a new patient Paul X during his initial visit was that in order to enter the trance state of hypnosis patients do not "go under" hypnosis. That is, he, as the subject would *"Go Iinto"* the hypnotic trance, rather than to going under my spell. Being overcome by the hypnotist's spell, I explained, was a definitive misconception of how hypnosis was performed. Within minutes of his 11 AM appointment Paul began questioning me, not only about the value of hypnosis, but of the entire procedure. He asked questions like:

- Was it possible he could not be hypnotized?
- What were my credentials?
- How would I put him under?
- Wasn't hypnosis harmful?

To resolve his skepticism about going into hypnosis and the process I would use, I pointed out my framed *American Board of Hypnotherapy* certificate, and my clinical hypnotherapy certification with *The American College of Hypnotherapy*. I also informed him that I offered a hypnotherapy certification course approved by the same college. Then, I explained that as the author of *The Trance Zone Hypnosis Manual*, and that I always abide by my mission statement developed many years ago. I recited it verbatim, *"Inspire The Injured Spirit And You Can Dissipate Any Disease."* Then I told him, honestly: *"Your spirit has been injured. Your mental state is unbalanced because you are infected with the disease called negativity."*

<u>Too Many People Are Skeptical About Hypnosis</u> (continued)

It wasn't long before I learned that this high-powered attorney, with over 25 years experience had been feeling like a terrible looser. He had been suffering with such low self-esteem that his upper lip twitched as he began describing his state of depression. His stuttering subsided only after he accepted my explanation that I would be guiding him with imagery and positive suggestions, and that HE and not the therapist would always be in control of the session. This misunderstanding was not uncommon for someone undergoing hypnosis their first time. He felt solace after I explained that all he had to do was open his eyes to terminate the session.

As the attorney sat dumbfounded in expression I consoled him, "You don't have to take my word for any of this. Just give me ten minutes. If you feel what we're doing together isn't working you can leave and there will be no charge. And, yes, we would be doing this together." So, this was not as if a power-hungry hypnotherapist was taking control here.

After a brief history of hypnosis and an explanation of the use of *"the hypnotic eye,"* in conjunction with breathing and counting down, the attorney submitted to his first hypnotherapy session. A full half hour later, with the attorney "coming out" opening his eyes and sitting up, I saw a renewed man. This was a transformed man who felt completely at ease, as compared to the man who first entered my office.

Armed with the *Surgeon General's Report on Mental Health*, the knowledge of the *DSM-IV diagnostics manual*, and my self-assured manner, Paul soon understood he was in good hands. Convinced of my professionalism, he did not hesitate to write out a check for the initial fee. Additionally, as I deliberately pointed it out to him, his lip no longer continued twitching. The real acknowledgement of a job well done came when he called me from outside a half hour later. In an unusually calm voice, he set up three consecutive appointments for the following weeks ahead! *(more about the DSM-IV Manual in Chapter 9.)*

POSITIVE SUGGESTIONS & AFFIRMATIONS (continued)

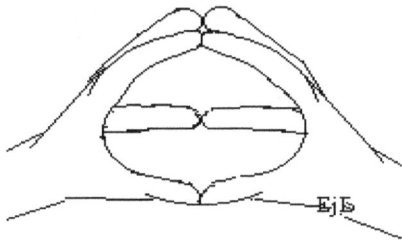

Illustration 8 – 1

Hypnosis Demonstration

Whether Hypnotherapist or Subject, this Hypnosis Demonstration should be very convincing in regard to testing the dominant powers of the subconscious over the conscious mind.

To Begin Place both hands together, spreading and placing the fingertips together, forming a hollow sphere. Focusing intently on the center while gently pressing the fingertips against each other, imagine a cylindrical fireball inside. Concentrate on having this fireball between your hands getting hotter, and hotter. As you feel the heat warming your hands press your fingertips together as hard as possible.

Then, while concentrating 100 percent on exerting full pressure, mentally think these words as you recite them audibly: "*I want to pull my hands apart*."
    Soon, you will discover that pulling them apart is physically impossible! The reason, being that you cannot exert two opposing forces in a positive direction. The lesson is that, where the positive force is strongest, the negative power becomes weakest. This is one of the best examples of how the subconscious can be programmed to overcome negativity, and yes, even illness.
    Find the positive force that overcomes the conflicting, negative weakness, and you have discovered the key to **positive transformation.**

When thoughts and words are said and done
There can always be room for improvement;
Whether in the bathroom or under the sun -
As long as it initiates positive inducement . . . EJL

POSITIVE SUGGESTIONS & AFFIRMATIONS (continued)

The Blue Aura Of Dharma Illustration (with the subject sitting or lying)

This is how you "Go Into" The Trance Zone, where only good things happen. In that wide opening to your subconscious, you are listening intently to my voice. You are sitting comfortably with your eyes still closed; your arms and legs are flexible, relaxed. Now, imagine yourself as being surrounded with a blue aura. And as you concentrate, this blue aura begins to glow more and more blue. Taking deep breaths let your entire body relax, but still keeping your arms in a comfortable, raised position.

Soon, while your blue aura continues to glow, it gets warmer and warmer until you feel a rush of energy surging throughout your body. This energy is a positive and healing energy; it is such a powerful energy it overcomes you to the point you feel a tremendous confidence in yourself. And, keeping this feeling of confidence know your self worth, know that you are loved and precious. Now, I would like you to relax all your muscles and let yourself become free of tension.

Let yourself be. Let whatever happens happen, because great things are taking place. Your mind is free of all worry, free of daily problems and headaches. As you sit, free of worry, you rejoice in the sense of well being that your blue aura brings to you, which envelops you from head to foot. Feel and experience this wonderful sensation which spreads more and more throughout your body.

You feel protected, secure and full of high esteem as the sensation forms a permanent place in your subconscious. Your subconscious is registering all my words. Wider and wider, this opening has become. The gentle words of my voice are becoming deeply engraved as you listen intently to my suggestions. You are listening very intently as I proceed with great care.

Now that you are a free spirit, capable of going anywhere you wish, unafraid doing anything you desire, I'd like you to imagine yourself flying on the back of a huge white eagle. Higher and higher, you soar freely among the clouds on those thick, soft, protective feathers. You are unafraid because you are fully protected by this eagle. You are happy, and delighted at being far away from planet earth, far away from reality, far away from the boredom and the burdens that go along with all your daily functions.

Then, focusing and returning to the world below know that you have permission to become anyone you wish to be, accomplish anything you wish to accomplish. With your newly formed identity, envision yourself as the person you always dreamed you could be.

POSITIVE SUGGESTIONS & AFFIRMATIONS (continued)

Hypnotic Induction for Empowerment:

HYPNOTHERAPIST: (the following could be recited on tape)

I'd like you to form "the hypnotic eye" by placing the thumb and forefinger of either hand together, and place your hand at your side. This is the eye to your subconscious, which puts you into The Trance Zone. Now, I'd like you to lift your "eyes up to the eyebrows" and, when you feel like it, let your eyelids close. Keeping your eyes up take in a " deep yawn" and recite: "This is how I go into The Trance Zone."

Very good -- that is how you "Go Into" The Trance Zone, where only good things happen. In that wide opening to your subconscious, you are listening intently to my voice. Your arms and legs are flexible, relaxed. While I begin <u>counting down</u> from 12 by 2's until reaching zero, <u>inhale through the nose</u>, and exhale through the mouth, relaxing your body more and more upon each lower count. 12 . . . 10 . . . 8 . . . 6 . . . 4 . . . 2 . . . Zero.

In that wide opening to your subconscious, you are listening intently to my voice. You are resting, calm, relaxed, your eyes are closed and your arms and legs are flexible. You are free of tension, nothing distracts you as you feel yourself being drawn along, breathing slowly, regularly. You are completely relaxed as you feel this wonderful peacefulness enveloping your being.

In this state of peace you acknowledge that opening to your subconscious. This opening grows wider, more and more. My words are settling into your subconscious, are taking root there. You now submit to the following commands: So far you have been using only a small fraction of your mind - your conscious mind. You have been using less then five percent of your true potential because of using only your conscious mind. Now, using the natural power of the subconscious, you are able to use more and more of your true power. Right now you have permission to use the total power of your subconscious mind. Every minute of every day your mind gets better and better in every positive way.   Every minute of every day, your mind continues developing to its fullest potential - even now, it now has become better in every possible way.

When I count to five you will open your eyes feeling alert and refreshed. Every part you will feel better than ever before. One . . . two . . . You feel alert and refreshed. Three . . . four . . . You are alert, and fully alive. Five . . . It's time to open your eyes.

Note: When performing a deep hypnotic trance always guide the patient into a healthy, present state using the typical "Come Out," as described above.

POSITIVE SUGGESTIONS & AFFIRMATIONS (continued)

To Instill Direction And Motivation

You call upon your creative powers in order to enable you to choose the right direction. You have the ability to concentrate on completing the project nearest your ideals, nearest your passion, your creativity, and your most deeply rooted inclinations. You now have the ability to summon the powers within you to motivate yourself. You now have enough motivation to become active in putting together your ideal project and completing it, concentrating on it day by day until you succeed.

Again, you have enabled the power within you to summon your innermost abilities to initiate your tremendous capacity for active energy. You have now initiated your total being in order that you heighten and manifest whatever powers are within you. You now feel very adequate and ready to accomplish that innate desire within yourself. In your mind's eye you already know you have what it takes to get this completed. You know all this is true, and you readily accept it.

Personal Magnatism

Personal Magnetism rules the world. In order for you to realize the power of this statement, you should know there are adjustments to be made in your life. Since everything indicates that great magnetic forces develop in persons who know how to purify their bodies through love and healthful living, it is to your enrichment to do the same. Beginning right now, agree to accept temperance in all things - from moderation in food consumption, to a simple diet, to strategic physical exercise, to calmness and kindness, to evenness of mind. This is already accepted subconsciously - it happened at the beginning of this induction, when I stated that Personal Magnetism rules the world.

As you go into that wide opening to your subconscious, know that all the traits of Personal Magnetism have been stored there. This enables you to make use one of the most powerful tools the mind can possess any time you wish. Between your newly acquired knowledge of Personal Magnetism, doors to every imaginable scenario are now being opened to you. Already, you realize that some people sense you are the spiritual person they have been looking for, that you are a caring person of deep knowledge, wisdom and compassion. Know that friends and even strangers may want to offer you money and other golden opportunities.

POSITIVE SUGGESTIONS & AFFIRMATIONS (continued)

The Divine Wish Conception

Imagine a decorative water fountain with statues pouring water into a pool at its base. See yourself standing in front of it with a sparkling coin in your hand. While you stare at the coin and make your finest wish, you imagine your guardian angel approaching you, giving you a blessing. As you toss the coin high in the air, keep your eyes glued to it; watch it hit the water until it settles to the bottom of the pool. Focusing on the coin, make it grow large enough to see what you wished for appear larger-than-life. Realize that if you believe strong enough, and have faith long enough, anything is possible.

To Refrain From Overeating

Willfully, you will go on a five day fast. You will loose all desire to overeat. You will eat very slowly and stop eating as soon as the feeling of "fullness" registers its message. Soon you will desire to begin some form of exercise. As you do so, listen closely to the instinctive messages your body sends you -- feel its true vibrations. Your natural instincts will tell you exactly what your weight should be, and will adjust accordingly. From this day forward, you agree to let your body be the judge of how much you should eat, and let your emotions stand aside. As of right now, this is your well-deserved reality.

To Overcome Illness

You are coming into a very deep subconscious state. Your imagination is free and clear. Here, you are enabled to use the power of your imagination to help you attain whatever it is you need to accomplish. I command that part of your subconscious that is responsible to restore your original powers. Now, you are enabled to begin functioning perfectly, just as you were intended to do from the beginning.

I address all the cells of your being, and command them to restore your powers. I call attention to your healthy cells and instruct them to heal you and make you healthy. These commands to your cells give them permission to begin your healing process. The healing process is already working and, in a very short period, the affects shall take place accordingly, and dramatically. Your natural instincts will tell you exactly what is needed and will adjust accordingly. From this day forward, you agree to let any negative attitudes stand aside. As of right now, this is your well-deserved reality.

POSITIVE SUGGESTIONS & AFFIRMATIONS (continued)

Overcoming Disease Cell by Wonderful Cell

Perhaps you already know that when you are in the deeply relaxed state as you are now, every nerve and every cell in your body is able to restore and rejuvenate itself. Deep within your subconscious, you know your body has the intelligence to heal itself, cell by wonderful cell, so that your organs improve and become healthier. When you are quiet and peaceful, as you are right now, realize that there is a part of you that knows what parts need restoration, and exactly what to do about it. Maybe you already noticed the increase throughout your immune system, and that your symptoms and ailments are disappearing. And you can continue to imagine, and accept that all the areas of your body that need healing are healthy, strong, and pure. Deep within you, you know that your subconscious knows exactly how to cure everything.

Journey Away To Your Vacation

After taking a safe flight, miles away from home, you find yourself riding in a convertible along the French Rivera. Since you have been enjoying the afternoon basking on the beach, you pull into special garden café where you know they go to extremes to please their patrons. While being led to a private wooded area, you become overwhelmed with your surroundings: beautiful weeping willows with colorful lanterns suspended high among them, while waitresses pass back and forth serving drinks along the adjacent pool.

And then you see the hammock being spread between the trees, especially for you. As you slip into the canvas with your full weight, you find yourself swinging side-to-side, smiling contently because you are being served your favorite juice. Suddenly, you realize everything is just as you always dreamed it would be.

Quitting Bad Habits (Or Other Addictions)

Through the practice of hypnosis, it is feasible to break a bad habit, which is a negative, degenerative habit. This is accomplished by replacing it with a good habit, which becomes a positive, beneficial habit. Everyone develops habits, but some are positive, while others are negative. The problems rise when our negative, or bad, habits control us - for they begin inducing demoralizing, and abusive, self-defeating traits. They are called "bad habits" because they are bad for us, personally, and sometimes just as bad for those around us. Whether falling into patterns of negative conditioning, or self-destruction – reprogramming harmful thoughts can be successfully used to alter the defeatist personality.

POSITIVE SUGGESTIONS & AFFIRMATIONS (continued)

To Overcome Insomnia (short version)

While your body has a tremendous ability to heal itself, the subconscious mind actually serves as the regulator of every possible part, every possible function. Not only does your subconscious have the ability to perform all the healing you need, it has the capability to initiate peaceful rest and sleep when called upon. To get to sleep, go deep into your trance and speak to your subconscious mind. Talk to it, just as if it has the power and understanding to listen to your requests – for it does, you know.

All you have to do is ask that you be given the opportunity to sleep when it comes time to retire for the night. Repeated often enough at bedtime, you will be granted your request. Remember that Desire, Belief and Expectation are very necessary tools. In combination with exercise and proper nutrition, as well as proper ventilation, you will learn to apply these in order to overcome your bouts with insomnia.

Your subconscious mind is capable of extraordinary recouping powers, and endless capacities, even while you enjoy your peaceful sleep. You <u>know</u> that, and you can continue to allow your body to rejuvenate while you relax and enjoy feeling peaceful. That deep place in your subconscious mind acknowledges all this and remembers to initiate sleep at bedtime. And even after you come out of this exhilarating trance state, you can trust your ability to initiate sleep whenever it is needed.

Note: As demonstrated in previous chapters, through the practice of Mind-Altering Suggestions, persons can actually become conditioned to alter their personality traits. Part of the hypnotherapist's obligation is to guide the subject into the trance state by offering helpful hypnotic suggestions, and by verbally painting colorful images, or guided imagery.

Aside from experience and creative talent, the hypnotherapist's WORDS are, perhaps, the most powerful of all the tools. Do not become disappointed if it doesn't seem the client will experience the trance - even though it is very likely. Hypnotherapy does take lots of Practice, Patience and Persistence - the three P's of any successful endeavor.

POSITIVE SUGGESTIONS & AFFIRMATIONS (continued)

9 Common Myths and Misconceptions
(Permission by James Mapes)

MYTH #1 Hypnosis is a mysterious magic power:
Hypnosis was accepted as a science by the American Medical Association in 1958. There is nothing supernatural or magical about hypnosis. The fear people have of hypnosis reflects lack of knowledge, fear of the unknown or prejudice.

MYTH #2 Only weak willed and unintelligent people can be hypnotized:
In truth, the opposite is true. The stronger the will and the more intelligent the easier it is for a subject to enter into "state". Everyone goes in to and out of a trance state many times a day: daydreaming, watching television, working at a computer, becoming so absorbed that you lose track of time, etc. Willingness, time, circumstances and the competence of the hypnotist are all factors in a person becoming hypnotized. I believe the ability to be hypnotized, or hypnotize yourself, is a skill. Some people have it naturally, like a child prodigy in music, and some need to practice in order to develop the skill. The majority of people fall in the latter category.

MYTH #3 A subject can enter a hypnotic trance, and not awaken:
Impossible! Impossible! Impossible! If you understand the concept of hypnosis, you will understand why. It's as ridiculous as believing a person can get stuck, forever, watching television. Even if the hypnotist were to walk away or drop dead in the middle of a show, the subjects would either open their eyes immediately or drift off into a normal sleep.

MYTH #4 People under hypnosis can be made to do things against their will:
Numerous studies have shown that participants will only act in a way that is congruent with their values and morals. People will only do, on stage, what they would normally do, given the right circumstances. Of course, people can be manipulated, lied to or coerced into doing things against their morals or values but you don't need hypnosis to do that.

MYTH #5 through #9 Continued Below:

9 Common Myths and Misconceptions (continued)

MYTH #5 Hypnosis will cause you to reveal your deepest hidden secrets:
This is one of the biggest fears that stop people from participating in the show. Hypnosis is not a truth drug which somehow breaks down the will of the subject. People, in a hypnotic state, always know what they are saying and what they are doing and will do nothing against their will or moral values.

MYTH #6 Hypnosis is in some way anti-Christian or the work of the devil:
This is the myth which creates the kind of fear which is hard to debate. The official view of the Catholic Church is that "Hypnotism is Licit if used for licit purposes:" (New Catholic Encyclopedia). All the other major religions have investigated hypnosis and approved it as a medical technique. And still, peoples' fear sometimes manipulates them in to believing hypnosis is something more than it is.

MYTH #7 When you are in a trance you are unaware of everything:
The word "trance" is confusing enough. Dictionary definitions of trance range from "a state of absorption" to "a stunned condition", from, "dazed" to "stupor." No wonder people are confused. Different people have different reactions to being in a trance state: Some people feel a sense of heaviness or lightness. Some people feel a tingling sensation and some feel nothing. The most important thing to remember is, in a trance state, you are aware of everything. In fact, your senses are heightened and your awareness is at a peak.

MYTH #8 Hypnosis can cure anything:
Hypnosis cures nothing nor is it a panacea. It is in the state of hypnosis where the real "magic" happens. With hypnosis you can *tap into your own power* to heal, manage pain, enhance creativity and athletic ability or eliminate negative habits. Hypnosis is, without a doubt, one of the most underutilized and powerful tools available for personal development. It can also greatly enhance your emotional and physical wellbeing.

MYTH #9 Hypnosis is dangerous and should be used by trained physicians:
Hypnosis is a tool of communication not medicine. Physicians practice medicine. Hypnotists practice hypnosis. Many physicians have embraced hypnosis and use it in pain control. Psychiatrists often use hypnosis in combination with psychotherapy.
The Only Danger of Hypnosis is The FEAR Some People Bring to It.

PART FIVE

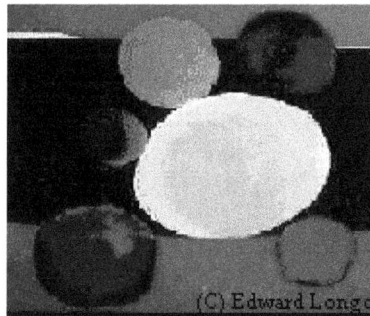

(C) Edward Longo

CHAPTER NINE
9

THE WONDROUS BRAIN
& THE DSM-IV

---

9 NEUROSCIENCE
MENTAL HEALTH:

Note: The following material is not intended to indicate being an authority on the entire workings of the mind, or the brain, for that matter (an irresistible pun). The information provided is solely to invite the hypnotherapist, practitioner, or other related professionals to become aware of the many ways they may gain access to vital knowledge, thereby becoming more helpful to mankind.

. . . the author, EJL

CHAPTER NINE
9

THE WONDROUS BRAIN
& THE DSM-IV

MENTAL HEALTH REPORT BY THE SURGEON GENERAL
The Fundamentals of Mental Health and Mental Illness

Excerpts from Library/Mental Health/Chapter 2: (References below)

A vast body of research on mental health and, to an even greater extent, on mental illness constitutes the foundation of this Surgeon General's report. To understand and better appreciate the content of the chapters that follow, readers outside the mental health field may desire some background information. Thus, this chapter furnishes a "primer" on topics that the report addresses. The report begins with a discussion of the brain because it is central to what makes us human and provides an understanding of mental health and mental illness.

All of human behavior is mediated by the brain.

Consider, for example, a memory that most people have from childhood - that of learning to ride a bicycle with the help of a parent or friend. The fear of falling, the anxiety of lack of control, the reassurances of a loved one, and the final liberating experience of mastery and a newly extended universe create an unforgettable combination. For some, the memories are not good ones: falling and being chased by dogs have left marks of anxiety and fear that may last a lifetime. Science is revealing how the skill learning, emotional overtones, and memories of such experiences are put together physically in the brain. The brain and mind are two sides of the same coin.

Mind is not possible without the remarkable physical complexity that is built into the brain, but, in addition, the physical complexity of the brain is useless without the sculpting that environment, experience, and thought itself provides. Thus the brain is now known to be physically shaped by contributions from our genes and our experience, working together.

This strengthens the view that mental disorders are both caused and can be treated by biological and experiential processes, working together. This understanding has emerged from the breathtaking progress in modern **neuroscience** that has begun to integrate knowledge from **biological** and **behavioral sciences**.

The Neuroscience of Mental Health
Complexity of the Brain I: Structural

As befits the organ of the mind, the human brain is the most complex structure ever investigated by our science. The brain contains approximately 100 billion nerve cells, or neurons, and many more supporting cells, or ganglia. In and of themselves, the number of cells in this 3-pound organ, reveal little of its complexity. Yet most organs in the body are composed of only a handful of cell types; the brain, in contrast, has literally thousands of different kinds of neurons, each distinct in terms of its chemistry, shape, and connections.

To illustrate, one careful, recent investigation of a kind of interneuron that is a small local circuit neuron in the retina, called the amacrine cell, found no less than 23 identifiable types. But this is only the beginning of the brain's complexity. The workings of the brain depend on the ability of nerve cells to communicate with each other. Communication occurs at small, specialized structures called synapses. The synapse typically has two parts. One is a specialized presynaptic structure on a terminal portion of the sending neuron that contains packets of signaling chemicals, or neurotransmitters. The second is a postsynaptic structure on the dendrites of the receiving neuron that has receptors for the neurotransmitter molecules.

The typical neuron has a cell body, which contains the genetic material, and much of the cell's energy-producing machinery. Emanating from the cell body are dendrites, branches that are the most important receptive surface of the cell for communication. The dendrites of neurons can assume a great many shapes and sizes, all relevant to the way in which incoming messages are processed. The output of neurons is carried along what is usually a single branch called the axon. It is down this part of the neuron that signals are transmitted out to the next neuron. At its end, the axon may branch into many terminals.

The usual form of communication involves electrical signals that travel within neurons, giving rise to chemical signals that diffuse, or cross, synapses, which in turn give rise to new electrical signals in the postsynaptic neuron. Each neuron, on average, makes more than 1,000 synaptic connections with other neurons. One type of cell—a Purkinje cell—may make between 100,000 and 200,000 connections with other neurons.

(continue)

The Neuroscience of Mental Health
Complexity of the Brain I: Structural (continued)

In aggregate, there may be between 100 trillion and a quadrillion synapses in the brain. These synapses are far from random. Within each region of the brain, there is an exquisite architecture consisting of layers and other anatomic substructures in which synaptic connections are formed.

Ultimately, the pattern of synaptic connections gives rise to what are called circuits in the brain. At the integrative level, large-and-small-scale circuits are the substrates of behavior and of mental life. One of the most awe-inspiring mysteries of brain science is how neuronal activity within circuits gives rise to behavior and, even, consciousness. The complexity of the brain is such that a single neuron may be part of more than one circuit.

The organization of circuits in the brain reveals that the brain is a massively parallel, distributed information processor. For example, the circuits involved in vision receive information from the retina. After initial processing, these circuits analyze information into different streams, so that there is one stream of information describing what the visual object is, and another stream is concerned with where the object is in space.

The information stream having to do with the identity of the object is actually broken down into several more refined parallel streams. One, for example, analyzes shape while another analyzes color. Ultimately, the visual world is re-synthesized with information about the tactile world, and the auditory world, with information from memory, and with emotional coloration. The massively parallel design is a great pattern recognizer and very tolerant of failure in individual elements.

The Neuroscience of Mental Health
Complexity of the Brain II: Neurochemical

Superimposed on this breathtaking structural complexity is the chemical complexity of the brain. As described above, electrical signals within neurons are converted at synapses into chemical signals which then elicit electrical signals on the other side of the synapse. These chemical signals are molecules called neurotransmitters. There are two major kinds of molecules that serve the function of neurotransmitters: small molecules, some quite well known, with names such as dopamine, serotonin, or norepinephrine, and larger molecules, which are essentially protein chains, called peptides. These include the endogenous opiates, Substance P, and corticotropin releasing factor (CRF), among others.

All told, there appear to be more than 100 different neurotransmitters in the brain. A neurotransmitter can elicit a biological effect in the postsynaptic neuron by binding to a protein called a neurotransmitter receptor. Its job is to pass the information contained in the neurotransmitter message from the synapse to the inside of the receiving cell. It appears that almost every known neurotransmitter has more than one different kind of receptor that can confer rather different signals on the receiving neuron. Dopamine has 5 known neurotransmitter receptors; serotonin has at least 14.

By definition, receptors that admit positive charge are excitatory neurotransmitter receptors. The classic excitatory neurotransmitter receptors in the brain utilize the excitatory amino acids glutamate and, to a lesser degree, aspartate as neurotransmitters. Conversely, inhibitory neurotransmitters act by permitting negative charges into the cell, taking the cell farther away from firing. The classic inhibitory neurotransmitters in the brain are the amino acids gamma amino butyric acid, or GABA, and, to a lesser degree, glycine.

Most of the other neurotransmitters in the brain, such as dopamine, serotonin, and norepinephrine, and all of the many neuropeptides constitute the second major class. These are neither precisely excitatory nor inhibitory but rather act to produce complex biochemical changes in the receiving cell. Their receptors do not contain intrinsic ion pores but rather interact with signaling proteins, called "G proteins" found inside the cell membrane. These receptors thus are called G protein-linked receptors. The details are less important than understanding the general scheme. Stimulation of G protein-linked receptors alters the way in which receiving neurons can process subsequent signals from glutamate or GABA.

(continue)

The Neuroscience of Mental Health
Complexity of the Brain II: Neurochemical (continued)

To use a metaphor of a musical instrument, if glutamate, the excitatory neurotransmitter, is puffing wind into a flute or clarinet, it is the modulatory neurotransmitters such as dopamine or serotonin that might be seen as playing the keys and, thus, altering the melody via G protein-linked receptors.

REFERENCES:
United States Department of Health & Human Services.
Office of the Surgeon General:

http://www.surgeongeneral.gov/library/mentalhealth/chapter1/sec1.html
http://www.surgeongeneral.gov/library/mentalhealth/chapter2/sec1.html
http://www.surgeongeneral.gov/library/mentalhealth/chapter2/sec1.html#complexity_2

CATEGORIZING MENTAL ILLNESS
Diagnostic & Statistical Manual of Mental Disorders, (DSM-IV)

Psychiatric Diagnoses are categorized by the Diagnostic and Statistical Manual of Mental Disorders, 4th Edition – (DSM-IV.) The manual is published by the *American Psychiatric Association* and covers all mental health disorders for both children and adults. It also lists known causes of these disorders, statistics in terms of gender, age at onset, and prognosis as well as some research concerning the optimal treatment approaches.

Mental Health Professionals use this manual when working with patients in order to better understand their illness and potential treatment and to help 3rd party payers (e.g., insurance) understand the needs of the patient. The book is typically considered the 'bible' for any professional who makes psychiatric diagnoses in the United States and many other countries. Much of the diagnostic information on these pages is gathered from the DSM-IV.

The DSM-IV manual is published by the *American Psychiatric Association*. Much of the information from the Psychiatric Disorders pages is summarized from the pages of this text. Should any questions arise concerning incongruencies or inaccurate information, you should always default to the DSM as the ultimate guide to mental disorders.

Diagnostic & Statistical Manual of Mental Disorders (continued)

What is Bipolar Disorder?

Bipolar disorder usually begins very early in life – it can sometimes start in early childhood, or as late as the 40s or 50s. When an adult over 50 has a manic episode for the first time, the cause is most likely to be a problem imitating bipolar disorder. Everyone has had ups, and downs, or mood changes of happiness, sadness, and anger at times. These generally are normal emotions and an essential part of everyday life. In contrast, however, bipolar disorder is a mental condition by which people have mood swings blown out of proportion, relative to things going on in their lives. These swings affect thoughts, feelings, physical health, behavior, and functioning. Bipolar disorder is not the result of a "weak," or unstable personality. Although this is a treatable disorder for which there are specific medications that can help, it is very probable that hypnotherapy will be able to play an important part regarding introducing positive, and sometimes permanent change.

The DSM uses a multi-axial or multidimensional approach to diagnosing because rarely do other factors in a person's life not impact their mental health. It assesses **five Axis dimensions** described below as:

Axis I: Clinical Syndromes
- This is what we typically think of as the diagnosis such as depression, schizophrenia, social phobia, etc.

Axis II: Developmental Disorders and Personality Disorders
- Developmental disorders include autism and mental retardation, disorders which are typically first evident in childhood.
- Personality disorders are clinical syndromes which have more long lasting symptoms and encompass the individual's way of interacting with the world. They include Paranoid, Antisocial, and Borderline Personality Disorders.

Axis III: Physical Conditions which play a role in the development, continuance, or exacerbation of Axis I and II Disorders
- Physical conditions such as brain injury or HIV/AIDS that can result in symptoms of mental illness are included here.

Diagnostic & Statistical Manual of Mental Disorders (continued)

Axis IV: Severity of Psychosocial Stressors

- Events in a person's life, such as death of a loved one, starting a new job, college, unemployment, and even marriage can impact the disorders listed in Axis I and II. These events are both listed and rated for this axis.

Axis V: Highest Level of Functioning

- On the final axis, the clinician rates the person's level of functioning both at the present time and the highest level within the previous year. This helps the clinician understand how the above four axes are affecting the person and what type of changes could be expected.

Diagnosing

There is a good deal of overlap among the different diagnoses listed in the DSM IV, which you may notice by browsing these pages. The reason for this is the same as for the overlap in medical diagnoses rarely is a symptom exclusive of anything, and rarely can a diagnosis be made without a pattern or cluster of symptoms. For example, Depression includes feelings of sadness, but anxiety can lead to sadness, as can phobias, psychosis, and many other disorders. Keep that in mind when reading about specific diagnoses or you may find yourself saying way too frequently "Oh my Gosh, I have that."

Diagnoses can only be made by a clinician (e.g., psychologist or psychiatrist) who specializes in these areas and who understands the symptom patterns and idiosyncrasies of each disorder. Don't self diagnose; if you feel you may have symptoms which are negatively affecting your life, please seek the advice and assistance of a professional.

Categories and Disorders

Mental Disorders are categorized according to their predominant features. For example, phobias, social anxiety, and post-traumatic stress disorder all include anxiety as a main feature of the disorder. All of these disorders are therefore categorized under Anxiety Disorders. For a complete listing of all disorders covered, use the Alphabetical Index. There's a lot of information there so please keep in mind that reading this information does not make you an expert in the nuances of mental health.

Diagnostic & Statistical Manual of Mental Disorders (continued)

EXAMPLE DISORDERS FROM THE DSM-IV Manual:

Major Depressive Disorder

Major depressive disorder features one or more major depressive episodes, each of which lasts at least 2 weeks (DSM-IV). Since these episodes are also characteristic of bipolar disorder, the term "major depression" refers to both major depressive disorder and the depression of bipolar disorder. The cardinal symptoms of major depressive disorder are depressed mood and loss of interest or pleasure. Other symptoms vary enormously. For example, insomnia and weight loss are considered to be classic signs, even though many depressed patients gain weight and sleep excessively. Such heterogeneity is partly dealt with by the use of diagnostic subtypes (or course modifiers) with differing presentations and prevalence. For example, a more severe depressive syndrome characterized by a constellation of classical signs and symptoms, called melancholia, is more common among older than among younger people, as are depressions characterized by psychotic features (i.e., delusions and hallucinations) (DSM-IV).

Psychiatric Disorders

Obsessive-Compulsive Personality Disorder
Diagnostic Criteria for Obsessive-Compulsive Personality Disorder
Obsessive-Compulsive Disorder (OCD)
Anxiety Disorders
Both biological and psychological causes have been found in OCD.

Symptoms

The key features of this disorder include obsessions (persistent, often irrational, and seemingly uncontrollable thoughts) and compulsions (actions which are used to neutralize the obsessions). A good example of this would be an individual who has thoughts that he is dirty, infected, or otherwise unclean which are persistent and uncontrollable. In order to feel better, he washes his hands numerous times throughout the day, gaining temporary relief from the thoughts each time. For these behaviors to constitute OCD, it must be disruptive to everyday functioning (such as compulsive checking before leaving the house making you extremely late for all or most appointments, washing to the point of excessive irritation of your skin, or inability to perform functions like work or school because of the disorders.

Diagnostic & Statistical Manual of Mental Disorders (continued)

Treatment

Medication is often prescribed for individuals with OCD. Psychotherapy can be helpful in learning ways to feel more in control, cope better with stressors, and explore the underlying issues associated with the obsessive thoughts.

Narcissistic Personality Disorder

Personality Disorders

Like most personality disorders, there are many factors that may contribute to the development of symptoms. Because the symptoms are long lasting, the idea that symptoms begin to emerge in childhood or at least adolescence is well accepted. The negative consequences of such symptoms, however, may not show themselves until adulthood.

Symptoms

The symptoms of narcissistic personality disorder revolve around a pattern of grandiosity, need for admiration, and sense of entitlement. Often individuals feel overly important and will exaggerate achievements and will accept, and often demand, praise and admiration despite worthy achievements. They may be overwhelmed with fantasies involving unlimited success, power, love, or beauty and feel that they can only be understood by others who are, like them, superior in some aspect of life. There is a sense of entitlement, of being more deserving than others based solely on their superiority. These symptoms, however, are a result of an underlying sense of inferiority and are often seen as overcompensation. Because of this, they are often envious and even angry of others who have more, receive more respect or attention, or otherwise steal away the spotlight.

Treatment

Treatment for this disorder is very rarely sought. There is a limited amount of insight into the symptoms, and the negative consequences are often blamed on society. In this sense, treatment options are limited. Some research has found long term insight oriented therapy to be effective, but getting the individual to commit to this treatment is a major obstacle.

Diagnostic & Statistical Manual of Mental Disorders (continued)

Narcissistic Personality Disorder (continued)

Prognosis

Prognosis is limited and based mainly on the individual's ability to recognize their underlying inferiority and decreased sense of self worth. With insight and long term therapy, the symptoms can be reduced in both number and intensity.

REFERENCE:
Diagnostic and Statistical Manual of Mental Disorders, 4th Edition, better known as the DSM-IV. The manual is published by the *American Psychiatric Association.*

STRESS and DEPRESSION

The stress response is important for survival and adaptation. The stress response, which involves both emotional and physiological changes, is an adaptive response that motivates our behavior so we can protect ourselves. It is turned on by the brain working in specific neural circuits modulated by neurotransmitters and hormones. There are important individual differences in humans. Some people may have the ability to quickly shut down their emotional, behavioral, and hormonal responses to stressful situations, while others may have prolonged responses.

While research funded by the National Institute of Mental Health (NIMH), part of the National Institutes of Health, has resulted in profound advancement in most of the major mental illnesses, in 2006 we recognize that not all treatments work for everyone. After six decades of progress mental disorders remain unacceptably common, causing more disability in people under age 45 than any other class of non-communicable medical illness. Over time, these prolonged responses could affect physiology and brain function. For example, increased release of cortisol over a long time could affect glucose regulation, bone density, immune function, and the function of specific brain cells. These individuals could become vulnerable to developing physical and mental diseases. Evidence suggests that over activity of corticotropin-releasing factor, a brain neurochemical, may play a role in why some people become excessively anxious and depressed. About 50 percent of depressed patients have over activity of the stress hormone response, which is regulated by corticotropin-releasing factor.

Stress and Depression (continued)

Whether this over activity causes or contributes to depression is unclear. It is also possible that over activity of this system may play a role in altering the structure and function of certain brain cells. Studies of childhood experiences may reveal a connection between stress hormone levels and depression. A study in 1945 by Spitz examined the psychological condition of orphans who were hospitalized and provided with a clean and healthy environment but with very little contact or comfort by the nurses

These children were described as withdrawn and social interactions with them became increasingly difficult. In more recent studies, data suggests that children who have been deprived of contact or comfort develop alterations in their stress hormonal responses. Studies of monkeys also can provide some insight into the relationship between stress hormones and depression. One long-ago experiment by Harlow focused on monkeys who were raised apart from their mothers with little or no physical contact with other animals. When these monkeys became mothers, they were either indifferent and withdrawn or violent and abusive to their offspring; they were unable to regulate their own emotions. This suggests that their early experience promoted the development of a vulnerability that proved to be very important when they became adults.

The offspring of these motherless mothers, moreover, began to exhibit similar abnormal behavior. The fact that some of the motherless monkeys were withdrawn and others were abusive reflects the differences among individuals who experience trauma. We can't give a complete answer as to why one individual responds in one way and another responds in a completely different manner. We're dealing with very complicated brain systems involving numerous brain chemicals interacting across many brain regions. Scientists hope that by studying how the stress response system relates to development and depression they may be able to develop early recognition and new treatment strategies, perhaps targeting early environmental factors as well as the hormonal systems that may be affected.

Mental Health Research: Into the Future:

In the six decades that NIMH has led the nation's research effort in mental health, advancement has been dramatic. We understand now that the major mental disorders are brain disorders, with specific symptoms rooted in abnormal patterns of brain activity. We realize that the devastation of autism and schizophrenia are not the result of bad parenting or early psychic conflict.

Mental Health Research: Into the Future: Stress and Depression (continued)

We recognize that mental disorders, unlike most chronic medical disorders, generally begin in childhood, with 50 percent of affected adults reporting onset of symptoms before age 14.

We now have reliable diagnostic tools as well as effective medications and psychological therapies for depression and anxiety disorders; we have treatments that can predictably reduce the hallucinations and delusions of schizophrenia, as well as psychosocial interventions that enable people with schizophrenia to remain in their communities, to work and lead productive lives. The number of patients in state hospitals has decreased from 600,000 to less than 60,000.

SOURCE: NIMH
http://www.nimh.nih.gov/about/dirupdate_researchfuture.cfm

NOTE: The information herein has been provided to increase knowledge and to gain a better understanding of hypnotherapy.

CHAPTER TEN
10

THE MARVELOUS AUTONOMIC SYSTEM

---

10 NERVOUS SYSTEM
PHYSIOLOGY:

__Autonomic Nervous System:__ The part of the nervous system that is responsible for control and regulation of the involuntary bodily functions, including those of the heart, blood vessels, visceral smooth muscles and glands: it consists of the sympathetic system, which in general, stimulates the body to prepare for physical action or emergency, and the parasympathetic system which, in general, stimulates the opposite responses.

__Autonomic:__ 1 - Occurring involuntary; automatic; 2 - of or controlled by the autonomic nervous system; 3 - Biology: resulting from internal causes, as through mutation

. . . New World Dictionary (p93)

__The autonomic nervous system__ is controlled mainly by the hypothalamus and is in turn divided into two sets of nerves: the sympathetic and parasympathetic nervous systems. Each of these two systems has a distinct anatomical location and communicates with its target organs through other neurons located in ganglia. Although the autonomic nervous system is considered to be involuntary, this is not entirely true. A certain amount of conscious control can be exerted over it as has long been demonstrated by practitioners of Yoga and Zen Buddhism.
(Review **The Brain** at http://www.thebrain.mcgill.ca/flash/index_d.html)

CHAPTER TEN

10

THE MARVELOUS
AUTONOMIC SYSTEM

ORGANIZATION OF THE NERVOUS SYSTEM
Autonomic and Sympathetic Nervous Systems

Autonomic Nervous System

The autonomic nervous system consists of sensory neurons and motor neurons that run between the central nervous system (especially the hypothalamus and medulla oblongata) and various internal organs such as the: heart, lungs, viscera glands (both exocrine and endocrine) It is responsible for monitoring conditions in the internal environment and bringing about appropriate changes in them. The contraction of both smooth muscle and cardiac muscle is controlled by motor neurons of the autonomic system.

The actions of the autonomic nervous system are largely involuntary (in contrast to those of the sensory-somatic system). It also differs from the sensory-somatic system is using two groups of motor neurons to stimulate the effectors instead of one. The first, the preganglionic neurons, arise in the CNS and run to a ganglion in the body. Here they synapse with postganglionic neurons, which run to the effecter organ (cardiac muscle, smooth muscle, or a gland.)

(continue)

Autonomic Nervous System (continued)
The autonomic nervous system has two subdivisions:
- *1 - Sympathetic nervous system,
- *2 - Parasympathetic nervous system.

*1 - Sympathetic Nervous System

The sympathetic nervous system goes into action to prepare the organism for physical or mental activity. When the organism faces a major stressor, it is the sympathetic nervous system that orchestrates the "fight-or-flight" response. It dilates the bronchi and the pupils, accelerates heart rate and respiration, and increases perspiration and arterial blood pressure, but reduces digestive activity. Two neurotransmitters are primarily associated with this system: epinephrine and norepinephrine. The preganglionic motor neurons of the sympathetic system arise in the spinal cord. They pass into sympathetic ganglia, which are organized into two chains that run parallel to and on either side of the spinal cord. The preganglionic neuron may do one of three things in the sympathetic ganglion: synapse with postganglionic neurons which then reenter the spinal nerve and ultimately pass out to the sweat glands and the walls of blood vessels near the surface of the body pass up or down the sympathetic chain and finally synapse with postganglionic neurons in a higher or lower ganglion leave the ganglion by way of a cord leading to special ganglia (the solar plexus) in the viscera.

Here it may synapse with postganglionic sympathetic neurons running to the muscular walls of the viscera. However, some of these preganglionic neurons pass right on through this second ganglion and into the adrenal medulla. Here they synapse with the highly modified postganglionic cells that make up the secretory portion of the adrenal medulla. The neurotransmitter of the preganglionic sympathetic neurons is acetylcholine (ACh). It stimulates action potentials in the postganglionic neurons. The neurotransmitter released by the postganglionic neurons is noradrenaline (also called norepinephrine).

The action of noradrenaline on a particular gland or muscle is excitatory is some cases, inhibitory in others. (At excitatory terminals, ATP may be released along with noradrenaline.) The release of noradrenaline stimulates heartbeat, raises blood pressure, dilates the pupils, dilates the trachea and bronchi, stimulates the conversion of liver glycogen into glucose, shunts blood away from the skin and viscera to the skeletal muscles, brain, and heart, inhibits peristalsis in the gastrointestinal (GI) tract, inhibits contraction of the bladder and rectum.

Autonomic Nervous System (continued)
*1 - Sympathetic Nervous System (continued)

In short, stimulation of the sympathetic branch of the autonomic nervous system prepares the body for "fight or flight" emergencies. Activation of the sympathetic system is quite general because a single preganglionic neuron usually synapses with many postganglionic neurons; the release of adrenaline from the adrenal medulla into the blood ensures that all the cells of the body will be exposed to sympathetic stimulation even if no postganglionic neurons reach them directly.

*2 - The Parasympathetic Nervous System

The activation of the parasympathetic nervous system causes a general slowdown in the body's functions in order to conserve energy. This is the mode is associated with the hypnotic trance due to its tendency to loosen up the muscles as well as slowing down the breathing. Whatever was dilated, accelerated, or increased by the sympathetic nervous system is contracted, decelerated, or decreased by the parasympathetic nervous system. The only things that the parasympathetic nervous system augments are digestive functions and sexual appetite. One neurotransmitter is primarily associated with this system: acetylcholine.

The main nerves of the parasympathetic system are the tenth cranial nerves, the Vegas nerves. They originate in the medulla oblongata. Other preganglionic parasympathetic neurons also extend from the brain as well as from the lower tip of the spinal cord. Each preganglionic parasympathetic neuron synapses with just a few postganglionic neurons, which are located near, or in, the effector organ, a muscle or gland. Acetylcholine (ACh) is the neurotransmitter at all the pre-ganglionic and many of the postganglionic neurons of the parasympathetic system. However, some of the postganglionic neurons release nitric oxide (NO) as their neurotransmitter.

Parasympathetic stimulation causes slowing down of the heartbeat, lowering of blood pressure constriction of the pupils, increased blood-flow to the skin and viscera, peristalsis of the GI tract. In short, the parasympathetic system returns the body functions to normal after they have been altered by sympathetic stimulation. In times of danger, the sympathetic system prepares the body for violent activity. The parasympathetic system reverses these changes when the danger is over. The Vegas nerves also help keep inflammation under control. Inflammation stimulates nearby sensory neurons of the Vegas.   (continue)

Autonomic Nervous System (continued)

*2 - The Parasympathetic Nervous System (continued)

When these nerve impulses reach the medulla oblongata, they are relayed back along motor fibers to the inflamed area. The acetylcholine from the motor neurons suppresses the release of inflammatory cytokines, e.g., tumor necrosis factor (TNF), from macrophages in the inflamed tissue.

Example 1: Sodium (Na) and Chlorine (Cl) = Ionic Bond. There is a large difference in electro-negativity, so the chlorine atom takes an electron from the sodium atom converting the atoms into ions (Na+) and (Cl-). These are held together by their opposite electrical charge forming ionic bonds. Each sodium ion is held by 6 chloride ions while each chloride ion is, in turn, held by 6 sodium ions. Result: a crystal lattice (not molecules) of common table salt (NaCl).

Example 2: Carbon (C) and Oxygen (O) = Covalent Bond there is only a small difference in electro-negativity, so the two atoms share the electrons Result: a covalent bond (depicted as C:H or C-H) atoms held together by the mutual affinity for their shared electrons an array of atoms held together by covalent bonds forms a true molecule.

Example 3: Hydrogen (H) and Oxygen (O) = Polar Covalent Bond moderate difference in electro-negativity, so oxygen atom pulls the electron of the hydrogen atom closer to itself Result: a polar covalent bond Oxygen does this with 2 hydrogen atoms to form a molecule of water Molecules, like water, with polar covalent bonds are themselves polar; that is, have partial electrical charges across the molecule may be attracted to each other (as occurs with water molecules)[Link to schematic] are good solvents for polar and/or hydrophilic compounds. [Link to a schematic of how water molecules dissolve a crystal of table salt (NaCl)] may form hydrogen bonds.

Reference: John W Kimbell
http://users.rcn.com/jkimball.ma.ultranet/BiologyPages/P/PNS.html

(continue)

Autonomic Nervous System (continued)

Electronegativity: The Affinity for Electrons.

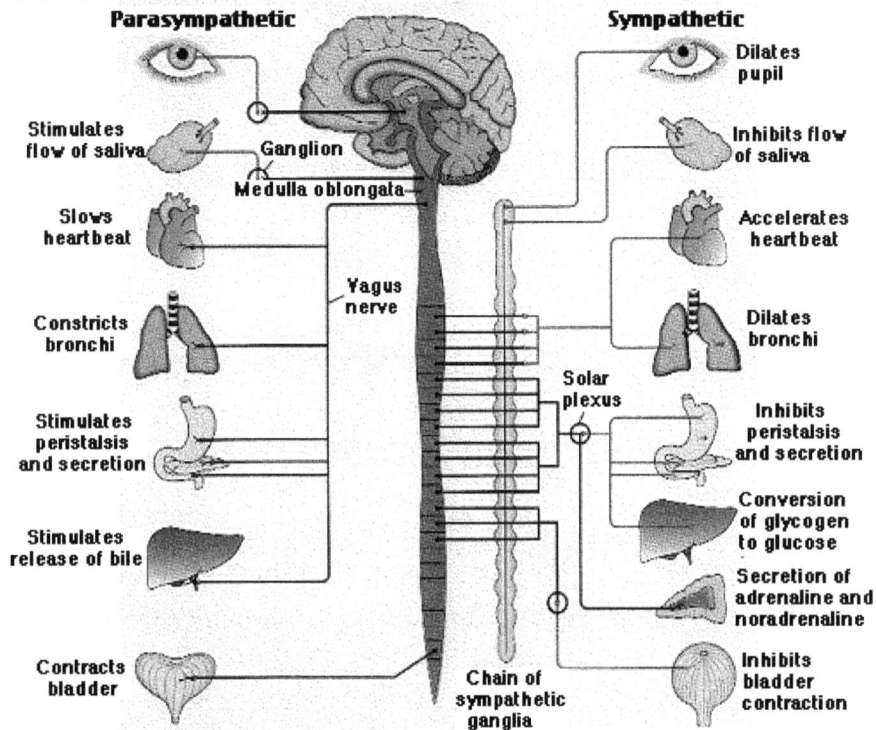

Autonomic Nervous System (autonomic.gif)

The atoms of the various elements differ in their affinity for electrons. This image distorts the conventional periodic table of the elements so that the greater the electro-negativity of an atom, the higher its position in the table. Although fluorine (F) is the most electronegative element, it is the electro-negativity of runner-up oxygen (O) that is exploited by life.

The shuttling of electrons between carbon (C) and oxygen (O) atoms powers life. Moving electrons against the gradient (O to C) – as occurs in photosynthesis – requires energy (and stores it). Moving electrons down the gradient (C to O) – as occurs in cellular respiration - releases energy.

The relative electro-negativity of two interacting atoms also plays a major part in determining what kind of chemical bond forms between them.

Reference: John W Kimbell

http://users.rcn.com/jkimball.ma.ultranet/BiologyPages/E/Electronegativity.html

Autonomic Nervous System (continued)

The Natural Pacemaker:

The heart has its own "electrical system." This system sends out signals that determine the heart's rate or rhythm. This is made possible by the unique properties of the muscle cells of your heart: they can contract and then relax in response to electrical stimulation.

A cardiac cycle ("heart beat") begins in the right atrium where very specialized cells form a small area called the Sinus Node (SA). The **Sinus Node** is also called the **pacemaker of the heart**, since it sets the pace or rhythm of your heart. The cells of the Sinus Node cause an **electrical chain reaction that fires** spontaneously approximately 70 times per minute, and spreads **across the atria**, much like ripples on the calm surface of a pond, resulting in contraction (closing) of the atria.

The electrical impulses flow (propagate) like a wave, travelling down the atria, causing them to contract. As the atria contract blood is pushed into the ventricles, the heart's primary pumping chambers. The electrical impulse then propagates on to the ventricles by passing through the **Atrioventricular Node (AV,)** called **the Bundle of His,** and right and left **branches into both ventricles.**

The AV node provides the only normal path for the **electrical impulse** to travel from the atria to the ventricles. The electrical impulse then travels down to the ventricles through a network of specialized muscle fibers. This network divides into even smaller **Purkinje Fibers** that the impulse throughout both ventricles. The impulse stimulates the ventricles, **triggering them to contract and pump blood.** You can feel this contraction when you take your pulse.

As Defined by the Monopril Learing System. (The Heart Manual)

Autonomic Nervous System (continued)

The Double Helix

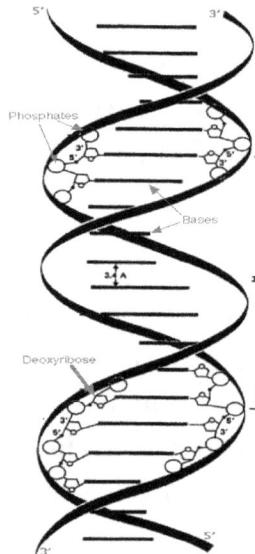

The double helix of DNA has these features: It contains **two polynucleotide strands** wound around each other. The backbone of each consists of alternating deoxyribose and phosphate groups (O-P-O). The phosphate group bonded to the 5' carbon atom of one deoxyribose is covalently bonded to the 3' carbon of the next. The **two strands are "antiparallel;"** that is, one strand runs 5' to 3' while the other runs 3' to 5'. The DNA strands are assembled in the 5' to 3' direction and, by convention, we "read" them the same way. The purine: Adenine (A) - Guanine (G)or pyrimidine: Thymine (T) - Cytocine (C) - Uracil (U) attached to each deoxyribose projects in toward the axis of the helix. Each base forms **hydrogen bonds** with the one directly opposite it, forming **base pairs** (also called nucleotide pairs, i.e. Base Paring).

Base Pairing

The double helix makes a complete turn in just over 10 nucleotide pairs, so each turn takes a little more (35.7 Å to be exact) than the 34 Å shown in the diagram. There is an average of 25 hydrogen bonds within each complete turn of the double helix providing a stability of binding about as strong as what a covalent bond would provide.

The diameter of the helix is 20 Å. The helix can be virtually any length; when fully stretched, some DNA molecules are as much as 5 cm (2 inches!) long. The path taken by the two backbones forms a major (wider) groove (from "34 A" to the top of the arrow) and a minor (narrower) groove (the one below).

Autonomic and Sympathetic Nervous Systems (continued)

Organization of THE LIMBIC SYSTEM

THE EMOTIONAL LIMBIC SYSTEM:

The structures listed below are often considered to constitute the limbic system. This system is involved in **olfaction, emotions, learning, and memory**. The limbic system was introduced as a concept by Paul MacLean in 1952 and was long considered the **seat of the emotions**. Though some of the structures included in this system are in fact involved in some emotional responses, we now know that it does not correspond exactly to any of the multiple emotional systems in the brain.

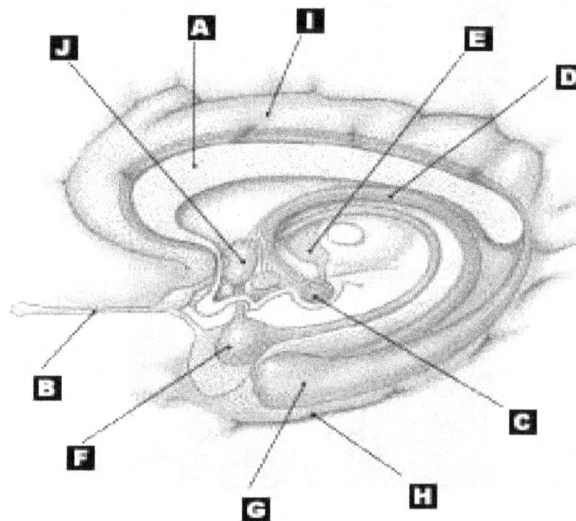

The limbic System (Paleomammalian Brain)
A- Corpus callosum, B- Olfactory tract C- Mammillary bodies,
D- Fornix, E- Anterior thalamic nuclei, F- Amygdala, G- Hippocampus,
H- Parahippocampal gyrus, I- Cingulate gyrus, J- Hypothalamic nuclei

RESOURCE:
http://www.thebrain.mcgill.ca/flash/a/a_01/a_01_cr/a_01_cr_ana/a_01_cr_ana.html#limbique

REFERENCES: John W Kimball
(http://users.rcn.com/jkimball.ma.ultranet/BiologyPages/B/BasePairing.html)
http://users.rcn.com/jkimball.ma.ultranet/BiologyPages/E/Electronegativity.html#covalent_bond
(http://users.rcn.com/jkimball.ma.ultranet/BiologyPages/N/Nucleotides.html)
(http://users.rcn.com/jkimball.ma.ultranet/BiologyPages/H/HydrogenBonds.html)

PART SIX

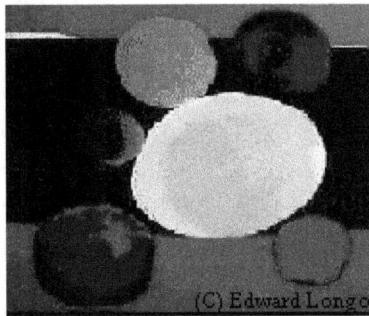

(C) Edward Longo

CHAPTER ELEVEN
11

MANIFESTATIONS OF THE
HIGHEST KIND

---

11 TRANSFORMATION
POSITIVE VISUALIZATION:

The hands in prayer can become a direct link between the subconscious and the supernatural and atomic forces of the universe. It IS possible to be transformed by the renewal of your mind that you may prove the perfect and complete will of God. This becomes obvious in the following quotation from the bible:

You will make your prayer to Him, and he will hear you;
And you will pay your vows.
You will decide on a matter, and it will be established for you,
And light will shine on your ways.
. . . Job 22: 27-28

CHAPTER ELEVEN
11

MANIFESTATIONS OF THE
HIGHEST KIND

TRANCE MANIFESTATIONS
Of The Highest Kind

Manifestations:
The forms in which someone, or something such as a person, a divine being, or an idea, is revealed; the materialized form of a spirit, or the discovery to the eye, or to understanding.

Of The Highest Kind:
Everything defined above, plus that which manifests, exhibits, or displays. Revelation: as in the Manifestation of God's Power in Creation.

In a documentary called The Ring of Fire shown on PBS television, they filmed a man actually igniting newspapers with the electricity produced from his bare hands and fingers. Sometimes when we pray, we place our hands together and, with great faith witness a miracle.

One of the basic understandings of the **Stanislavski Method** of acting is that the fingertips can be developed to such a degree they can become the actor's eyes. In **"Method"** acting, this serves to extend the actor's emotions and kinetic senses. To the blind person, the fingertips record the Braille and transform the meanings directly into visual images. With the use of the hands the blind are, sometimes, capable of sensing what emotions are coming through - merely by touching the person's face.

<u>TRANCE MANIFESTATIONS</u> (continued)

In demonstrating the powers of transformation, I cite the following example of metamorphosis: A larva produced by the caterpillar develops its cocoon from its worm-like pupa stage. Suddenly, one morning at the dawning of light, it transforms from its larva into its imago and manifests into an amazingly colorful, flying insect. Through a natural, though somewhat mysterious process called metamorphosis, the caterpillar has transformed into a Monarch butterfly. This is, perhaps, the most dramatic example of transformation, in that the physical body has become completely changed. But remember: Its **spirit** has also been changed in the process. It is not surprising that it flies thousands of miles, freely demonstrating its colorful, black and orange wing patterns.

Obviously, we are not about to change our bodies completely - but we can change everything else about us by virtue of self-improvement, especially by renewing the **spirit**. This can be accomplished with creative mind-body techniques, using the hands to heal patients of physical and mental disorders. Used in concert with hypnotherapy, great strides can be accomplished within the mind-body research community, and other areas of mental health.

Going Into **The Trance Zone** brings about an altered state of consciousness whereby, as if by some mystical power, the whole psyche shifts into an exaggerated state of positive exuberance. It is similar to that of **"the Zone"** that athletes talk about when an inner force takes over and places the participant into a state where every movement seems effortless. Tennis players and runners call it **"the second wind"** where every challenge seems a breeze; every, barrier becomes an invitation to a winning frame of mind. In other words, there is a surge of energy where everything, remarkably, falls into place. These remarkable states of euphoria could also be referred to as **"Success Zone."** or **"Pure Enjoyment."**

There is also another relative element that should automatically come into play in order to achieve positive transformation – it is the element of **"Positive Visualization."** Many successful people, especially those involved in sports activities, and especially those who are involved in the Olympics, have learned that focusing on visualizing the action prior to the actual event can often make the difference between success and failure.

(continue)

TRANCE MANIFESTATIONS (continued)

Below is a perfect example of what being in *"the Zone,"* or experiencing the, *"Pure Enjoyment"* mode, or **arousal state** can produce.

Sweet Sixteen Hughes edges Slutskaya, Kwan for gold - Press Release

SALT LAKE CITY (AP) - Posted: Thursday February 21, 2002
Another American teen-ager is wearing the Olympic gold medal that was supposed to belong to Michelle Kwan. Sarah Hughes, with the performance of her young life, soared from fourth place to win the free skate and the title Thursday night in one of the biggest upsets in Olympic figure skating history.

While Hughes played the same role as Tara Lipinski four years ago, Kwan made two major mistakes to fall to third, behind Russian Irina Slutskaya, who won the silver medal. Shortly after her routine, Sarah Hughes admitted it was the finest performance of her career. *"I skated for pure enjoyment,"* the 16-year-old Hughes said. *"That's how I wanted my Olympic moment to be."*

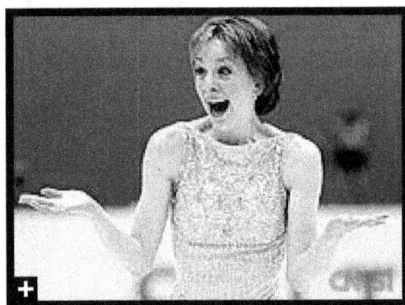

Illustration 12 -1
Sarah Hughes 2002 Gold Medalist

As coincidental as this may seem, just one week before completing this book I woke up reciting, 'I am the power of the storm - I am the quiet calm within the eye.' Well, here is what was most remarkable about this: In noticing my left arm was somewhat raised, I had become surprised to find I had awakened with my left hand forming "The Hypnotic Eye." And, believe me, I had not been practicing this related to sleep, at all. This was actually how I came to include it in the hypnotic trance script located below. Talk about positive visualization . . . EJL

Note: One of the basic understandings of the Stanislavski Method of acting is that the fingertips can be developed to such a degree they can become the actor's eyes.

TRANCE MANIFESTATIONS (continued)

Alchemy: A method or power of transformation; especially the seemingly miraculous change of a thing into something else. - *New World Dictionary*

The hypnotherapist, as alchemist, can prepare to enhance the power of the hands by massaging them in a special way: First massage the fingers, one-by-one, increasing the blood flow; then slowly press each hand backwards at the wrist, loosening the tension; next, flip the hand over and pull each finger inside toward the wrist, loosening up the muscles and tendons. Finally, interweave the fingers, squeezing and manipulating the hands until all the joints become free of tension - and then rub the hands together, stimulating them. Prior to, or during, the session it would be helpful to perform Mesmer passes or, if the client is willing, apply hands-on healing exercises touching the head, neck, or solar plexus. Eventually, recite the following trance script:

HYPNOTHERAPIST - AS ALCHEMIST
HYPNOTHERAPIST
Have the subject *"Go Into"* <u>The Trance Zone</u> as follows:
I'd like you to form "the hypnotic eye" and place it at your side. This is the eye to your subconscious. Now, I'd like you to lift your "eyes up to the eyebrows" and, when you feel like it, close them. Keeping your eyes up, take in a "deep yawn." Very good – that is how you "Go Into" <u>The Trance Zone,</u> *where only good things happen. As I begin counting down from 12 by 2's, I'd like you to "inhale through the nose" and exhale through your mouth. 12, 10 . . . Good, breathe slowly and calmly. 8, 6 . . . That's right, inhale through your nose. 4, 2 . . . Zero.*

This radiant, pure light within you is energizing and transforming your spirit that miracles are taking place mentally, physically and emotionally. This inner, illuminated light has created within you a sound mind and body, and is curing you of all disease and disorders. As you concentrate think only of tranquility as you continue to breathe deeply, steadily, and evenly. As you listen to my voice, you are confident, having the knowledge that you are in good hands.

Know that I am here to activate, stimulate and rejuvenate all the elements of your whole being in mind, body and spirit. Concentrate on this knowledge as you breathe deeply, having the incoming oxygen replenish your entire immune system, your entire being. Know that my energy is flowing through me to you, in order that you become well. Know this, believe it, and accept it as a divine gift to you coming from above.

HYPNOTHERAPIST AS BEHAVIORIST
Behavior Modification

Behavior Modification: A technique that seeks to modify animal and human behavior through application of principals of conditioning, in which rewards and reinforcements, *or punishments (not practiced in hypnotherapy)* are used to establish desired habits, or patterns of behavior. - *New World Dictionary*

The hypnotherapist, as behaviorist, may advance the practice of hypnotherapy by understanding the techniques animal trainers use to modify the behavior of dogs, and other pets. It would also be helpful to spend time watching trainers of circus elephants, horses, and even tigers. The study of pussycats can also provide lessons on behavior – especially in the way they focus, and how they are able to stretch and relax. There are many other ways to understand behavior including watching the activity of strangers, or waiters, or observing social gatherings.

As far as incorporating change during the hypnosis session, the hypnotherapist must have a keen insight as to what the client may need in order to make the transformation as positive, and as permanent as possible. Some people are able to do this intuitively, while others must practice and study human behavior on multiple levels, perhaps multicultural as well.

ANOTHER EXAMPLE INDUCTION – DEEP STATE
HYPNOTHERAPIST
Have the subject *"Go Into"* <u>The Trance Zone</u> as follows:

I'd like you to form "the hypnotic eye" and place it at your side. This is the eye to your subconscious. Now, I'd like you to lift your "eyes up to the eyebrows" and, when you feel like it, close them. Keeping your eyes up, take in a "deep yawn." Very good – that is how you "Go Into" <u>The Trance Zone</u>, where only good things happen. As I begin counting down from 30 by 2's, I'd like you to "inhale through the nose" and exhale through your mouth. 30, 28, 26, 24, 22, 20 . . . Good, breathe slowly. 18, 16, 14, 12, 10 . . . Just let your body relax. 8, 6, 4, 2 . . . Zero.

In that wide opening to your subconscious, you are listening intently to my voice. You are lying comfortably. Your eyes are closed. Your arms and legs are flexible, relaxed. Continue breathing evenly, inhaling through your nose and exhaling through your mouth. With each breath, you sink deeper and deeper and deeper into a relaxed state of mind. You no longer want anything.

(continue)

ANOTHER EXAMPLE INDUCTION – DEEP STATE (continued)

Become passive as you listen to my voice. Let yourself go. Let it be . . . Let it happen. Nothing bothers or distracts you. Nothing bad or unusual is going to happen. Your head is clear. Your mind is free of all problems. You rejoice in this sense of peace and wellbeing that envelops you from head to foot. Feel this wonderful relaxation, which spreads more and more throughout your body. Feel the new looseness and weightlessness of your body. In this wonderful state of peace, you have an opening to the subconscious - wider and wider this opening is becoming.

Your subconscious is registering all my words. The gentle words of my voice are being deeply engraved there as you listen intently to my suggestions. You are listening very intently as I proceed with care. Good, breathe slowly and calmly.   Let your body relax more and more each time. Relaxing, relaxing, going deeper and deeper into hypnosis. As you are resting comfortably, you will notice that your eyes are closed tight, very tight. They are stuck so tight you are not able to open them. Your eyes are stuck together so tight they feel as if they are sealed with a mudpack.

In that wide opening to your subconscious, you are listening intently to my voice. Perhaps you already know about your subconscious mind's extraordinary powers of self-healing, and how the right side of your brain controls the functioning of your entire body.

The right side of your brain, the subconscious mind, knows how to regulate your breathing even while you are sleeping, and knows how to regulate your circulatory system, how to carry the right nutrients to all the parts of your body that need them. This brilliant part of your mind also knows how to instruct every cell in your body to heal itself, to improve, to feel more comfortable and to be healthy and sound, cell by cell. And I don't know how fast your body is healing itself now, but your mind knows just how to accelerate the healing that is already taking place in your body. Yes, your subconscious has the intelligence and the power to heal anything inside of you on an intercellular basis.

You may have read or heard, or perhaps you know from your own experience that athletes need to take great care in order for their bodies to grow strong, and recuperate from overwork. And as you rest your body now, like an athlete rests, your body can become stronger and healthier, revitalizing your nerves, your blood, and even your brain cells. And although the aging process is always causing deterioration, it doesn't have to follow that your vision, your memory or your legs have to become weakened.   (continue)

ANOTHER EXAMPLE INDUCTION – DEEP STATE (continued)

And I don't know if you have already felt certain sensations in your body, signaling that the healing process has already started, but you can be sure that while you are in this deep, resting trance state, your body is already healing itself. You can enjoy feeling relaxed, knowing your body can accelerate and improve your immune system even now, as you enjoy this rest. Know for sure that you can rely on your inner self; that you can count on that part of you in your subconscious that knows exactly what to do, and exactly how to do it.

Perhaps you remember a time when you had a cut that was so deep you felt it wouldn't heal, or perhaps you had a bout with the flu. You probably went to a doctor for treatment, but then even as you slept and played and worked, your body did all the healing. While your body has a tremendous ability to heal itself, the subconscious mind actually serves as the regulator of every possible part, every possible function. Not only does your subconscious have the ability to perform all the healing you need, it has the capability to initiate peaceful rest and sleep when called upon. Your subconscious mind is capable of extraordinary recouping powers, and endless capacities, even while you enjoy this peaceful state.

You know that, and you can continue to allow your body to rejuvenate while you relax and enjoy feeling peaceful. That deep place in your subconscious mind acknowledges all this and remembers the need to recall everything when we are through. And even after you come out of this exhilarating trance state, you can trust your ability to initiate peace and relaxation whenever it is needed. When you go to bed at night, you take delight in the fact that sleeping serves to replenish your entire body, hour after hour, cell by remarkable cell.

Imagine every part of your body *becoming so relaxed it seems like jelly. Allow this liquid tranquilizer to relieve every pain, every arthritic condition, every restrictive feeling in you body.   Allow this tranquilizer to balance your entire nervous system, your complete immune system, as you focus on allowing your mind to come to complete rest. You are free of all worry, free of all tension as you drift off into your hypnotic trance. Deeper and deeper you go into this deep trance state; deeper and deeper you go into hypnosis. The deeper you go into hypnosis, the deeper you go into this trance state. Deeper and deeper, you drift off into your beautiful, restful hypnotic trance.*

(continue)

ANOTHER EXAMPLE INDUCTION – DEEP STATE (continued)

In order that your dreams become fulfilled, listen carefully as I plant these thoughts deep within that brilliant, manifestation compartment of your mind. As far as love goes, that wide opening to your subconscious is now open to receiving love, along with all the touching, embracing and sharing that goes along with it. Through the supernatural powers above, you are now capable to allow and accept love in every form. You are now open to receiving love from the special compatible person or persons you have been longing for. Now, love is able to flow into your life, enough so that it will fulfill all your romantic and sexual needs; enough that you receive love more readily, and expeditiously than ever before.

Now that you have closed your eyes, I would like you to focus on your breathing while I continue giving you positive suggestions, and guided imagery. Still concentrating on your breathing, make sure you continue to inhale through your nose and exhale through your mouth. Going deeper into hypnosis while listening to my voice allow your breathing to calm all nervousness, or tension. And, with your eyes still closed, please gently squint and relax them, and then focus on the colors inside your eyes. Now squint your eyes again and notice the changes. That's very good - now relax and go deeper into hypnosis.
As you continue breathing deeply and calmly, you know in your heart that your ideal state of mind is that of calmness and tranquility. In this peace that encompasses your whole being, you feel almost as if time has stopped. All worries are put aside, all tension and pain has left your body. In that wide opening to your subconscious, you feel you are in complete control of the healing powers of your own immune system, as well as all your vital organs. In this state of tranquility, your subconscious mind prevents any disease from disrupting your mental or physical health.

Now, with your hand forming "The Hypnotic Eye," I would like you to repeat this after me: I am the power of the storm; I am the quiet calm within the eye. Very good - bear in mind that "quiet" means dismissing noise, and that calm means total relaxation physically, as well as emotionally. Please be assured that while you go even deeper into hypnosis every problem will become resolved. Know that all issues regarding your stress and anxiety have become diminished to the point you have a tremendous confidence in yourself. This information will stay with you even after you arise from this all empowering trance.

HYPNOTHERAPIST AS BEHAVIORIST

7 SECRETS OF ATTRACTING LUCK

"If it be not now, yet it will come. Being ready is all." . . . *William Shakespeare.*
In other words:
"If it is not already here, it will come – being ready is everything." . . . EJL

As described all throughout this book, you already possess the power of releasing the unlimited potential within you. By applying the principles contained in this book, you already possess the key to unlocking the doors that have held you captive. The only limitations are those which lie within the mentality of the person creating, or denying them.

The **7 Secrets Of Attracting Luck** have been revealed so that you may have a full understanding of what it takes to develop a sound mind and body, as well as to reverse bad luck, or to turn chance into opportune luck. They are listed below in the order of prioritization. The first thing to do is to establish a **Method** of approaching the issue. Then, muster the **Motivation** to apply **Meditation** and **Matriculate** it by altering the **Mentality** and acquiring **Magnetism**, and in time, things will **Manifest** far beyond your wildest expectations.

But, before beginning to apply the knowledge of these secrets, follow the procedures as described below. First, learn to focus on hands, either with the eyes open or closed. Lift the hands above the head and run them down your body to get the feel of how your illuminated light affects you. Then, imagine the subject you wish to influence and focus, applying positive thoughts regarding the desired outcome, whether to mesmerize, or bring change.

However, before expecting to receive the appropriate outcome, you must first learn to apply the **7 Secrets Of Attracting Luck.** For example, to have the number become lucky for you, hold the hands over a sheet of paper with the **Number 7 enlarged.** Then focus on that number, influencing it with positive thoughts of winning money, or becoming **Lucky** in various other ways.

7 SECRETS OF ATTRACTING LUCK (continued)

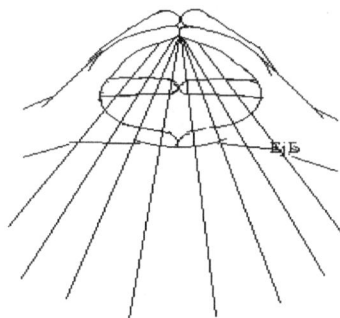

Illumination Therapy ™
Illustration 12 –2

"You will decide on a matter,
and it will be established for you,
and light will shine on your ways."

Study, apply, and practice the 7 Secrets Of Attracting Luck as listed below and, before you know it, a life filled with fortunate experiences will manifest before you – in real life. Then concentrate on drawing supernatural power from above while reciting: *Since I am through with facing poverty, Infinite riches are flowing freely into my life. Each and every day I am growing more and more prosperous.*

While doing this, visualize as vividly as possible, money floating down, surrounding you with fifty and hundred dollar bills. In applying this concept as instructed, I'm sure you will agree that the possibilities are endless.

1. **Method** – As explained above, the most important thing to do is to develop and practice your own way to focus on the sphere, pulling in laser-like, illuminated light from the universe. Everyone has a plan or an idea of how to become a winner, but only those who have a way of tapping into the universal powers become truly successful at it. For success does not just mean wealth, but also the gratification, self-esteem and integrity gained from following ones pureness of heart. There may be other methods of finding true mastery over fate, but it may be difficult to find anything as powerful as the above, **Illumination Therapy ™**.

(continue)

7 SECRETS OF ATTRACTING LUCK *(continued)*

2. **Motivation** – There are many ways to become motivated. The question is which motive works for **you**; what does it take to get **you** to feel the spark and the drive to accomplish your objective? Believe it or not, the four D's: Disposition, Discipline, Dexterity and Determination have a great deal of impact on whether or not you receive positive results. For example, your Disposition has a lot to do with your attitude, your frame of mind, your mood, in that it effects your drive to become a winner. Once you acquire the Discipline to take control of your destiny, you will find that things begin to fall into place. Your Dexterity, on the other hand, has much influence on the way you comprehend the road ahead of you. Above all, you must acquire enough Determination to firmly set your course, whether by committing to decisions, or by setting strong enough objectives that will inspire you to become motivated.

3. **Meditation** – You can definitely influence the outcome of your fate through the power of **Mind-Altering** affirmations, or prayers. Or by inducing hypnotic suggestions such as: *Like a special friend, I am looked after and supported by my higher spiritual power and the special forces of the universe in all areas of my health, wealth and relationships.* You will find many more ways of acquiring the powers of meditation through the practice of hypnotic suggestions, mind-altering affirmations, and prayers.

4. **Matriculate** – In order to penetrate the part of subconscious mind, which is responsible for producing good luck, *"Go Into" The Trance Zone* and ask to receive the proper guidance regarding your requests. Ask for the right answers to your dilemmas, or how you can turn <u>chance</u> into <u>opportunity</u>. Whether fortune, health, or love be your aspirations, it's all there, waiting to be called upon. All you have to do is tap into your source.

5. **Mentality** – One of the important keys to receiving good fortune is the mind-set, the mental attitude, or mode of thinking. When focusing with an optimistic heart, together with child-like enthusiasm, nothing seems impossible – therefore the possibilities of successful outcomes become something inherent. Misfortune, or unfortunate experiences, commonly associated to being "bad luck" irrefutably stem from conditions that instill fears. With a sincere attempt to become introspective, begin to examine the possible masks of fear that might have been affecting your attitude – fears that actually serve in draining positive energy. The list of masks that cause fear is extensive, the major ones being as follows: anger; jealousy; lust; ego; aggressiveness; depression; possession; obsession; prejudice; over-protectiveness; smothering; insecurity; judgment; unhappiness and dissatisfaction. All of these fears interfere with our natural elements, from love to supernatural existence. At this juncture, you may ask, what doesn't consist of fear? Love, spiritual faith, and loyalty to God – that's about the best.

(continue)

7 SECRETS OF ATTRACTING LUCK (continued)

6. **Magnetism** – At the fore, spiritual harmony with the universe, better understood as charisma, is the most effective way to generate attraction. Because Personal Magnetism rules the world, and since everything indicates that great magnetic forces develop in persons who know how to purify their bodies through love and healthful living, it is to your personal embellishment to participate accordingly. To begin with, try inducing hypnotic suggestions such as: *Like a magnet, with special compelling attributes, I attract good fortune and abundance in my life. Since abundance is my natural state of being, I readily accept it now.*

7. **Manifest** – Manifestation is a remarkable phenomenon, a source governed by luck. **Good luck** is based on harmony, not discord; organization, not chaos; capability, not inadequacy: shrewdness, not stupidity; relaxation, not tension; anticipation, not hindsight; resolution, not procrastination; decisiveness, not doubt; trust, not disbelief; and finally, it is based on acceptance, not denial. With a keen eye – whether focusing on monetary, physical physiological, or spiritual power – you can finally look forward to **Manifestations Of The Highest Kind**. Of all the forces on earth, luck still prevails as one of the most powerful, good or bad. Given in the information above, as well as the descriptions below, the secrets to good luck have been revealed to you. All you have to do now is apply them. Since the number **7** is considered **lucky**, I have included it under that number. But remember that the thought of having anything become lucky is only as good as its positive conception, where the unprecedented optimistic reaps the rewards of being a formidable winner. The **Formula** for **Luck** is described below . . . **Good luck**.

(continue)

7 SECRETS OF ATTRACTING LUCK (continued)

LUCK – The Formula:

Leverage the possibilities. Nurture your advantages for all their worth. Play your cards, but know when to fold them. Sometimes it might better to take quick, small loss, rather than to chance a drawn out, large loss. After all this information is computed, acknowledged and incorporated, the chances are that you will become lucky enough to amass great wealth -- but remember this: millionaires have no real freedom. They are too busy holding onto to their money, investing it, and therefore becoming enslaved to it. So, be careful of what you ask for, because you are very apt get it.

Ultimately follow goals to completion. Many years ago, sometime in the early 1900's, a little known writer came up with the notion that he could write a good story about a girl and her dog. The two became entrapped in a cyclone, and then became carried into another time, another land, where the girl would meet three very odd people. He had great faith in this story, although it was just a children's story. I suppose he hoped that it would become published, but the author didn't write for the money, or the success -- he wrote because he loved his work with a **passion**. It was something that **motivated** him; gave him **purpose** – he **needed** to create. His name was L. Frank Baum, and that children's story became so popular it was turned into that famous movie called, *The Wizard Of Oz*. Yes, the road to his success definitely became paved with a yellow, brick road – which actually became his road to gold.

Calculate the risks and Commit to them. Speaking of roads, that illusive road to success has been paved with many a failure. Yet, without taking calculated risks, there can be no great gains. Since the difference between success and failure is similar to the difference between winning and losing, we are always focused on the struggle between them. It is there that the chance of becoming lucky, or not, comes into play. In realizing that, the ability to increase the odds of winning becomes, not only based on the manner in which the calculations are made, but in the determination to commit to those calculations.

Ken is a rarely used word encompassing a wide range of Knowledge. **Ken** not only encompasses an understanding beyond one's self, its meaning, in addition to vision, is comprised of cognizance and mental perception. Without considering all the aspects of **Ken**, making the proper calculations would leave the individual seeking **luck** incapable of drawing the proper conclusion. Every bit of gathered information must be analyzed and scrutinized before making any kind of decision regarding the **lucky**, or unlucky, aspect of the deduction. For example, considering the four elements that could go wrong when betting on horseracing – the quality of the horse; the attitude of the jockey; and the condition of the track – betting would be fruitless if either of these elements were miscalculated. What about whether the horse was running on the outside rail, or whether it had experienced a muddy track before? Here, the use of **Ken** would certainly make a difference: understanding, vision, cognizance, and mental perception.

<u>7 SECRETS OF ATTRACTING LUCK</u> (continued)

<u>LUCK</u> is not made – it is thought up; envisioned good, or bad!
Being in the right place at an opportune time also has a lot to do with luck. But, in being at that place at the particular time can be brought about by keeping an open line to those universal laws. The late millionaire, Howard Hughes, being stranded in the desert, once promised a man over a half million dollars for lending him a quarter, merely because he stopped the car to pick him up. Was this coincidence, or chance? Or was it because of the man's giving nature. "Give, and you shall receive," is but one element of that universal law. To insure that good luck will manifest itself, I have added the final letter **<u>Y</u>**, and its definition to the equation, as listed below.

<u>Y</u>es, I am lucky -- Emblazon these words in your mind.
As an attempt to demonstrate the kind of perception it takes to make a proper calculation, I cite the following bit of information only as an example as to concept.

On Easter Sunday of this year, a publicist friend of mine invited me to dinner at Ben's Restaurant in New York City. While being introduced to the owner, I happened to notice the giant-sized horseshoe hanging on the wall. Since I already knew how greatly successful the restaurant had become, I asked Ben, the owner, whether it made any difference whether the horseshoe was hanging upside down, or not. To my surprise, I learned that it <u>did </u>make a difference – his response was that the horseshoe must be hung with its legs turned upward in order to **attract luck** and **hold it inside**. Armed with this kind of <u>knowledge</u> (**<u>Ken</u>.**) whether suspicious in nature, or not, a person would be better equipped to draw the proper conclusion and proceed accordingly.

All good luck is based on desire, belief, and expectation. The key being: neither to allow negative influence from without, nor to entertain negative thoughts from within. *Playboy's* Hugh Hefner got what he wished for – his vast fortune began with a solitary wish from the wishing well right on his property when he was still poor. He became **lucky** because he **desired**, **believed**, and **expected** his wish to come true. In essence, by having great faith in the powers that be, he enabled innate good fortune, already within him, to manifest itself.

In conclusion, using every means possible, make sure you <u>apply</u> the key words: **Desire**, **Belief**, and **Expectation**. Congratulations, you now possess the most powerful tools ever developed to attract **good luck**. Now you can prepare yourself for that winning streak you've been yearning for. By the way, it is the culmination of **<u>Ken</u>** and its key elements, which actually bring about winning streaks. The rest is in your hands.

Now, because of your **Determination**, you have learned what it takes to become **Lucky**.

Congratulations . . . **<u>LUCKY!</u>**

CHAPTER TWELVE
12

INDUCING
MAJESTIC TRANCE SPELLS

---

12 SELF-HYPNOSIS
CONDITIONING:

*Of all
the **negative forces** that
undermine the subconscious mind
Defeatism
Depression, and **Deprivation**
are among the most damaging to the
physiological makeup,
as well as to
the emotional psyche.*

. . . EJL

CHAPTER TWELVE
12

INDUCING
MAJESTIC TRANCE SPELLS

MAJESTIC TRANCE SPELLS
Through Self-Hypnosis

Although spells are though of as being of the occult in origin the trance spells presented in this chapter are essentially methods of intense focus in order to arrive at a positive subconscious trance. The purpose of initiating the varied trance spells herein is simply a way of utilizing concentration, or focus, so that they may serve as empowerment, verses any kind of negative hocus pocus.

Due to the fact that it is not immediately recognizable, depression is the primary cause of self-abuse, insomnia, addiction and the consequences of rejection. It is also responsible for inferiority complexes, phobias and obsessive compulsion disorders, as well as an entire spectrum of other maladies. Because most victims of defeatism become so caught up in their problems, they become unaware of these influences - they have become blinded to their own inability. In affect, they become powerless and succumb to the dominant forces sabotaging their subconscious. The old saying, "You can't see the forest through the trees" has some truth in it. If you wish to see the big picture, you need to advance and examine the layout of the forest.

The following **Majestic Trance Spells** will aid in resolving the distress, negativity, and doubt caused by deprivation. To augment the **Majestic Trance Spells**, try placing a small multifaceted crystal, or transparent marble, between the fingers to represent *"The Hypnotic Eye,"* Visualizing the object, and then closing the eyes and feeling its effect, will aid in deepening the hypnosis. When going into the trance, simply focus and imagine being empowered by a divine, mysterious eye within the fingers.

Focus on **Majestic Trance Spells** listed below, creating vivid images in your mind whenever possible. In time, and it could be sooner rather than later, the answer to your problems will become realized. To enhance your subconscious powers, even further, practice **The Seven Day Trance Spells,** and **Dream Fulfillment During Sleep** as described below. Soon, your desires, as well as your grandest dreams will manifest before you. Concentration, Conditioning, and Imagination are your newly found keys to prosperity and positive transformation.

SELF-HYPNOTIC SUGGESTIONS

Since the trance scripts below are designed to induce divine intervention, light up some Mt. Shasta sage, or frankincense during the ritual, and then focus on attaining the desired results. Prayers, beforehand, will help to produce results that may become even more effective. Tape record your Majestic Trance Spells then, whether the subject, or patient, "*Go into*" *The Trance Zone*, and listen to the selected message. To insure long-term results, they should be listened to twice every day under self-hypnosis for a period of at least two weeks. Please note that the trance scripts below are incomplete, and were mainly added to give the hypnotherapist ideas for creating audiotapes for clients. Therefore, with all the information gathered thus far, there should not be a problem with adding additional material according to the issues, or needs of each individual.

To Resolve the Siege of Deprivation and Defeatism

*Although I do not fully recognize it, negative forces have infiltrated my attitude, sabotaging my ego. Nothing is like what it should be, my finances, my love life, my social affairs, my health and my personal relations – all are suffering, and I do not know the cause. To rectify my situation, I will first change my attitude to that of being completely positive in all my undertakings. From now on my key WORDS are "**can do**." This means that any time I have doubts about my ability, or tasks at hand, I simply form "The Hypnotic Eye" and recall the WORDS, "**can do**." Doing this will instantly place me in a positive frame of mind.*

The next thing I need to do is change my behavior patterns. Therefore, I commit myself to making the firm decision to lift my spirits. I commit myself to positively improving my eating habits; cutting down on smoking; praying and meditating; and expressing and receiving love. I also commit to treating myself to things like an occasional movie; participating in group relations; participating in some form of exercise; or listening to uplifting music frequently.

Finally, I see the light. In order to alter this infliction that has caused me grief and pain, I resolve to participate in some form of behavior modification practice. Only then, will I be able to rectify my situation of being deprived of the essential things in life. Life should consist of things like self-gratification, expression, acceptance, good healthy stamina, and prosperity - not deprivation. And now, through the commitments ahead of me, I can see a direct path to inevitable happiness. My subconscious acknowledges my commitment, and has already planted the seeds to see all this through.

To Skyrocket The Power Of The Mind

I am resting, calm - relaxed. My eyes are closed and my arms and legs are flexible. I am free of tension, nothing distracts me as I feel myself being drawn along, breathing slowly, regularly. I am quite relaxed as I feel this wonderful peacefulness envelop my being. In this state of peace, I have an opening to my subconscious. This opening grows wider, more and more. My words are settling into my subconscious, are taking root there.

I now submit to the following commands: So far, I have been using only a small fraction of my mind, my conscious mind. I have been using less then five percent of my true potential because of using only my conscious mind. Now, using the power of the subconscious, I use more and more of my true power -- now, I am using the full power of my subconscious mind. Every minute of every day, my mind is better and better in every positive way. Every minute of every day, my mind continues to develop to its fullest potential - even now, my mind is better in every possible way.

To Modify And Cleanse The Mind

To enable me to initiate mind clarity, I now clear my mind of all negative and mentally harmful thoughts. I further clear my body of all illness, infection, and degenerative disease. And, I further clear my spirit of all evil forces and influences. I know that I have something more valuable than money – I have my health, my values, my good nature, and my loving, winning attitude. Since my body is the temple of the Lord, Jesus Christ, my subconscious recognizes that I am, indeed, God's property. This, my subconscious acknowledges, and through the powers that are majestic and supernatural, I have just modified, and cleansed my entire personality.

To Become Totally Optimistic

As I continue to focus on The Trance Zone, *I know that potential not faults enable me to become successful at whatever I choose to do. I know that, by now, I am more appealing, more magnetic as far as my personality is concerned. I know that good fortune is on the brink, and yes it is due me. From this moment on, I deserve all the good things that will come my way. To put poetically: In my life there are things I need to know, so I condition myself to the seductive; while keeping the doors closed on things bad, opened doors guide me subconsciously -- insuring that I remain productive.*

To Attract Love Or A Mate

Every minute of every day, I'm getting closer and closer to meeting the mate who will be compatible, and good for me. Day by day, in every way I become attractive to the opposite sex. From this day forward, my best self is on the lookout for my compatible partner. Beginning right now, things are taking place to ensure that I will meet and "score" with a mate of my liking - with that person responding to me in kind, beginning right now. This process has already taken place and is being carried out through the power higher than myself. Subconsciously, I know and expect that this special matchmaking is taking place. I also know that this induction process is helping me to feel loved. I have come to realize that everything of true worth comes through love. This state of relaxation and utter trust has inspired me to grow as a person. It has allowed me to reach a privileged state of being loved, as well as being capable of loving.

To Become Sexually Appealing

In order for me to reach my highly magnetic, erotically appealing state, I take in deep breaths while I recite aloud: I am physically attractive to the opposite sex. My subconscious mind knows I have what it takes to be attractive. And it knows how to make the right adjustment to instill me with charm and magnetism. I feel this happening, right now. I feel it. I am a fitting, attractive person who is capable of reciprocating love and one so groomed that I make heads turn. As I keep taking in deep breaths through my nose and exhaling, repeating these words aloud, I know I have developed the energy and spark necessary to attract a mate. I am physically attractive to the opposite sex. My subconscious mind knows I have what it takes to be attractive. And it knows how to make the right adjustment to instill me with charm and magnetism. I feel this happening to me, right now.

To Attract Good Fortune

Realizing that being lucky is more than chance; I know how to improve my odds. By arming myself with the elements of positive decisiveness, preparation, focus, and expectation, I know that I improve my chances of becoming lucky. My advantage is in knowing that being lucky is not simply due to luck – it is due to the combination of these elements unfolding at precisely the right times. Being lucky means being skillful at anticipating when pulling these four elements together. By adding prayer, I have become a winner – because now I have five luck-inducing elements. I know life consists of things like gratification, expression, acceptance, healthy stamina, and prosperity. And, through the commitments ahead of me, I can see a direct path to my happiness. My subconscious acknowledges this, and has already planted the seeds to see all this through.

To Influence Lady Luck

*Every minute of every day, I get better and better in every way. Day by day, I get psychologically sound in every possible way.   As I accept this wholeheartedly as truth my thinking is sound, my behavior is sound - so quite naturally, my mind, body and spirit are now fully sound. As I focus on imagining the brightest star, I summon it to transmit winning vibrations through my body, down into the earth, and back within me to charge me with its most mystical powers. As I continue to focus, these powers supercharge me with unyielding lucky energies that actually influence everything I do. The more I focus, the more I become lucky, and the more I become lucky, the more I become a winner at everything I tackle; and that includes health, wealth and the pursuit of happiness. I feel this influence now. To enable Lady Luck to smile upon me, I invoke her to flow through me as I joyously begin humming the musical tune, **Luck Be A Lady Tonight.**

To Alleviate Arthritis

My neck and shoulders are more relaxed. As I relax more and more all the muscles surrounding, my neck and shoulders are looser and looser. My body processes are more efficient and my blood and tissue fluids now act to carry the impurities and wastes out and away. I feel this process relieving the clogging in my joints, relieving all my pain. As I concentrate on my shoulders, a drop of lubrication is secreted, loosening the joints of my neck and shoulders. Immediately, I feel the improvement and continue to feel better, healing more and more with every passing minute. I am pleased at this progress of recovery and have lost all desire to accommodate my arthritis. In that wide opening to my subconscious, I acknowledge that I have lost all susceptibility to arthritic symptoms.

To Strengthen The Mind, Spirit, And Immune System

As of this moment, I feel I am being released from all illness. I feel the energy of my mind, spirit and body, including my immune system, working at reversing my condition. As I keep breathing deeply and slowly, I can begin to feel my illnesses being transformed into the state of "wellness." I feel my misplaced energies of nervousness, apprehension and hostility subsiding, reacting to my breathing. Through the power of my subconscious mind, my sick cells have been transformed into positive, recuperative energies. The more I focus on deep breathing, the more dramatically my subconscious continues to cure me of all disease, and the aches and pains, as well as mental and physical stress.

THE SEVEN DAY TRANCE SPELLS

Since the following **Trance Spells** vary in scope, they should be individually incorporated into your standard self-hypnosis routine. However, at the end of each week, combining and taping them as one hypnotic session can produce amazing results. It may be helpful to tape the "Go Into," and "Come Out" portions of these scripts if deciding to record them as a weekly induction.

Sunday:
To Achieve Your Heart's Desire

I believe in myself and in the Higher Power that resides both in my mind and in the mind of the eternal one above. I call upon the Eternal One to enter these proceedings for we are One, One Power, One Universal Energy, myself being a channel through which this Power can flow. I believe in this Power, united through me, that guides all our lives. What man has done, I can do with the Eternal One working through me, because, knowing that I believe in this, I believe that all things are possible. My greatest desire at this time is to have all my hopes and dreams become fulfilled. To bring this situation about, my subconscious deep within me reassures me that I can, not through my will, but through Thy Will. It is done through the Universal Energy running through me; I repeat: It is done!

Monday:
To Improve Health And Fitness

Realizing from my own experience that athletes need to take care in order for their bodies to grow strong, or recuperate from overwork, they must have proper rest. Even as I rest my body now, like an athlete rests, my body can become stronger and healthier, revitalizing my nerves, my blood, and even my brain cells. And although the aging process is always causing deterioration, it doesn't have to follow that my vision, my memory or my legs have to become weakened.
And, since I already feel certain sensations in my body, signaling that the healing process is already started, I can be sure that while I am in this deep, resting trance state, my body has begun to heal itself. I can even enjoy feeling relaxed because of knowing my body can accelerate and improve my immune system even now, as I enjoy this rest. Through the power of my subconscious, I know for sure that I can trust your inner self, know that I can trust that part of my subconscious mind that knows exactly what to do, and exactly how to do it.

(continue)

THE SEVEN DAY TRANCE SPELLS (continued)

Tuesday:
To Become Totally Optimistic:

*As I continue to remain in **The Trance Zone,** I know that potential, not faults enable me to become successful at whatever I choose to do. I know that, by now, I am more appealing, more magnetic as far as my personality is concerned. I know that good fortune is on the brink, and yes it is due me. From this moment on, I deserve all the good things that come my way. To put poetically: In my life there are things I need to know, so I condition myself to the seductive; while keeping the doors closed on things bad, opened doors guide me subconsciously – insuring that I remain productive.*

Wednesday:
To Skyrocket The Power Of The Mind

I am resting, calm; relaxed. My eyes are closed; my arms and legs are flexible. I am free of tension, nothing distracts me as I feel myself being drawn along, breathing slowly, regularly. I am quite relaxed as I feel this wonderful peacefulness envelop my being. In this state of peace, I have an opening to my subconscious. This opening grows wider, more and more. My words are settling into my subconscious, are taking root there. So far, I have been using only a small fraction of my mind. I have been using less then five percent of my true potential because of using only my conscious mind. Now, using the supernatural power of the subconscious, I use more and more of my true power. Now, I am using the full power of my subconscious mind. Every minute of every day, my mind is becoming better and better in every positive way. Every minute of every day, my mind continues to develop its fullest potential in every possible positive way.

Thursday:
To Instill Direction And Motivation

I call on my creative powers in order to enable me to choose the right direction. I have the ability to concentrate on completing the project nearest my ideals, nearest my passion, my creativity, and my most deeply rooted inclinations. I now have the ability to summon the powers within me to motivate myself. Now, I am motivated to become active in putting together my ideal project and completing it, concentrating on it day by day until I succeed. Again, I have enabled the power within me to summon my innermost, tremendous energy. I have now initiated my total being in order to achieve whatever it is that is within me, and to accomplish that innate yearning within myself. In my mind's eye, I already know I have what it takes to get this completed.

THE SEVEN DAY TRANCE SPELLS (continued)

Friday:
To Gain Infinite Riches

Personal Magnetism rules the world. In order for me to realize the power of this statement, I know there are adjustments to be made in my life. Since everything indicates that great magnetic forces develop in persons who know how to purify their bodies through love and healthful living, it is to my enrichment to do the same. Beginning right now, I accept temperance in all things -- from moderation in food consumption, to a simple diet, to strategic physical exercise, to calmness and kindness, to evenness of mind. This already has been accepted subconsciously -- it happened at the beginning of this induction.

As I go into that wide opening to my subconscious, I see that all the traits of Personal Magnetism have become stored there. This enables me to make use one of the most powerful tools the mind can possess, and I have access to it any time I wish. Between my newly acquired combination of Magnetism and Hypnosis, doors to every imaginable scenario have become opened to me. Already, I realize that some people sense I am the spiritual person they have been looking for, that I am a caring person of deep knowledge, wisdom and compassion. Even now, I know friends, strangers and even my enemies want to do favors for me, as well as offer me money and other golden opportunities. Anything and everything can virtually become mine for the asking. The ease with which I am able to influence those around me to gain love, admiration, opportunities and wealth may seem amazing, but all the above became possible through the powers of Magnetism and Hypnosis -- the process of which I am participating in at this very moment. All is love, and love is everything. I thank God for the infinite riches flowing into my life.

Saturday:
To Induce Overall Healing

My subconscious mind has extraordinary intelligence when it comes to self-healing. It has the intelligence to heal anything inside of me on an intercellular basis. This brilliant part of my mind also knows how to instruct every cell in my body to heal itself, to improve, to feel more comfortable and to be healthy and sound, cell by incredible cell. The right side of my brain that controls the functioning of my body knows how to regulate my breathing even while I am sleeping. And it knows how to regulate my circulatory system, how to carry the right nutrients to all the parts of your body that needs them. Because my subconscious mind knows how to recall that it was my body that ultimately healed me cell by incredible cell, it knows exactly how to accelerate the healing – this healing that has already started taking place in my body.

DREAM FULFILLMENT DURING SLEEP

The standard practice regarding dreams was to attempt to interpret them after they have occurred. However, to my surprise, I have discovered that if a person would set up a **Dream Fulfillment** request prior to going to sleep, that request would become actualized during the dream state. Then, upon awakening, the person would be able to recall everything the dream revealed.

The request could be as simple as asking for a solution to a specific problem, or asking to live an experience that would bring a certain kind of fulfillment; sexual or financial gratification, for example. As you can imagine, this technique could produce richly rewarding results, having a remarkable, positive effect on one's welfare and self-esteem. Go into a trance and discover the Genie within you. Whether calling upon your spirit-guide, visionary, mediator, or a God - Ask, Seek, Knock and You Shall Find.

This is how it works: Prior to going to sleep, *"Go Into" The Trance Zone* and state your **Dream Fulfillment** request orally. Be as creative and as imaginative as you wish, instructing the subconscious to acknowledge your desires, and to enable you to recall them upon awakening. In believing, wholeheartedly, that your requests will be carried out during your dream state, the subconscious will act accordingly and manifest them, recording them as though they were real occurrences. After you awaken, just form *"the hypnotic eye"* and you will recall everything. The beauty of this technique is that you will have experienced the entire dream just as if it were real, giving you the fulfillment of even your wildest dream, since the subconscious cannot discern imagined truths from reality. Talk about benefits.

If your **Dream Fulfillment** request is too complex to memorize, tape it, then listen to it at bedtime. Remember that softness, directness, and clarity produces the best results. You probably will not be successful in the first few attempts. The more you believe in the process, the more effective it will become. To recall the dream after awakening it will be helpful to *"Go Into" The Trance Zone* and review what the subconscious recorded.

Finally, still concentrating on *"the hypnotic eye,"* ask your subconscious to reveal what was envisioned during your dream.

Listed below, is a **Dream Fulfillment Request** form. It is designed to build self-esteem, as well as to develop a formidable confidence in your imagery abilities.

Example:

To Enable Seduction (to be revised if female)

Form *"the hypnotic eye,"* and recite, (or record) the following trance script called *Dream Fulfillment Request* and play it at bedtime, or another convenient time (except when driving): *This is how I "Go Into" The Trance Zone, where my dream fulfillment request is resolved. In that wide opening to my subconscious ear, I acknowledge my dream fulfillment request as follows: As I approach my dream state, my subconscious mind creates images of me having sex with a beautiful woman. Because this lovely blond woman cannot resist my magnetism, she undresses herself, then me, and presses her lovely breasts against my naked body. Then she climbs on top of me and presses me firmly between her kegs. She kisses me frugally as she seduces me, nibbling and breathing into my ears until we both reach our climax. In my subconscious mind, I take note and record the seductive experience, to be recalled as soon as I awaken. I can also repeat this experience, whenever so desired.*

(If a woman, replace the words accordingly)

EXAMPLE: Dream Fulfillment Request Created by _____

(Write down your request and memorize it prior to going to sleep.)

Imagine how it would be to receive an Oscar at the Academy Awards. Set up the entire scenario, including tight shots and forming *"the hypnotic eye,"* prior to going to sleep. Remember, that concentration, focus, firm belief, and practice are always paramount in achieving any seriously intended results.

My Dream Request: ---

PART SEVEN

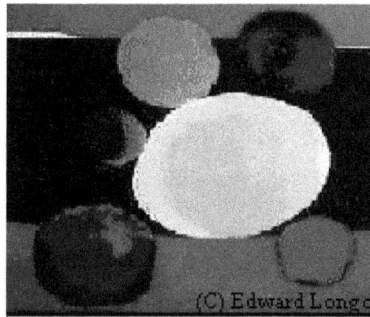

(C) Edward Longo

CHAPTER THIRTEEN
13

THE PHYSIOTHERAPY
TECHNIQUE ™

---

13 HYPNOTHERAPY
PHYSIOTHERAPY

Leonardo de Vinci once said to his disciples:

_"The soul does not like to be without its body
because without its body it cannot feel or do anything;
therefore build a figure in such a way that its pose
tells what is in the soul of it."_

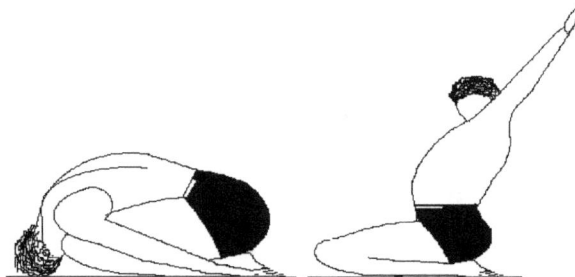

(C) EJL 1998

CHAPTER THIRTEEN
13

THE PHYSIOTHERAPY
TECHNIQUE ™

THE PHYSIOTHERAPY TECHNIQUE™
HEALTHY BODY; SOUND MIND; POSITIVE SPIRIT

Tending to mental and physical health has always been a constant struggle. If a person doesn't stick to a sound exercise routine and beneficial nutritional regimen, that person's body will tend to deteriorate before its time. For instance, if a person were to eat nothing but white bread, salt and coffee with loads of sugar, that person's body would soon become prone to disease and stroke. Add to this, alcohol and cigarette addiction, and the situation becomes even bleaker. On the other hand, if a person were to eat fish and an assortment of fresh fruits and steamed vegetables that person's body and vital organs would tend remain fruitful.

My explanation for this is that, from birth, nature's role is to see that we are given the opportunity to develop, spiritually, but mentally and physically, as well. After a time, when going against nature's role too long, the body begins its swing toward fatality. Think of it as the "degenerative swing." The principle is much the same as when an apple grows on a tree. After it falls, or is shaken off, the degenerative process begins to set in because its lifeline – its umbilical cord to nature – has been cut. Then, comes the rotting. Fortunately, as humans, we are blessed with the possibility, through nutrition and exercise, of decelerating this inevitable swing.

Through a never-ending responsibility to ourselves, we must see to it that our bodies get the proper exercise and nourishment, enough so that it becomes a sustaining fuel – a progressive blood / cell regeneration process. This physical conditioning is our only way of retarding the inevitable pull towards death. In fact, in the animal kingdom the expression "survival of the fittest" is truly representative of their way of life. In their world, the weak are always the first to succumb.

(continue)

THE PHYSIOTHERAPY TECHNIQUE™ (continued)

Physiotherapy

Ironically, it is the same in our world: "inevitable death" holds a ringside seat and continues to beckon the underdog called "self-neglect," while lasting life, the opponent as "the fittest," spars to claim the title of **longevity**. The exercises listed below are not only intended to improve the quality of life for those willing to participate, but they also insure that total fitness includes a sound mind, healthy body and a positive spirit so as to serve as that corridor to long life.

Consider the following The Physiotherapy Technique, if you will, as your free long-term, personal insurance policy. In this bowed praying position, bless yourself with the sign of the cross. Then begin meditating with various prayers in the position demonstrated in **Illustration 14 - 1**, below.

When appropriate *"Go into"* *The Trance Zone*, and proceed with the inductions that follow. It is a good habit to memorize the following prayers, reciting them audibly with the eyes closed, or by reading the scripts and meditating with the eyes opened. An additional benefit to crouching with the head down is that it sends blood and oxygen to the head and neck region, thereby replenishing brain cells, as impossible as it may seem. This will be more likely to happen with deep breathing.

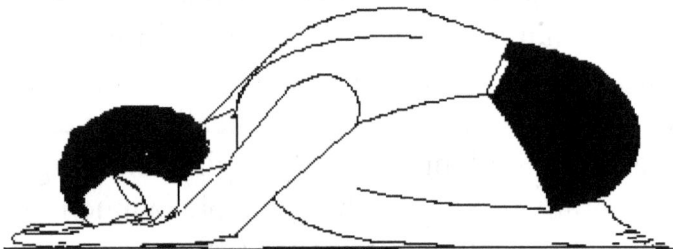

PRAYER POSITION
Illustration 14 – 1

While crouched in this special Prayer Position practice meditating on trance inductions such as listed below. Since the eyes must be open to allow reading the trance scripts, consider practicing the *"Go into"* *The Trance Zone* technique so that the meditative state will become deeper. Or, try reciting and then listening to a prerecorded tape with the eyes closed. Since sounds resonate through neurotransmitters, affecting the glands and organs, playing inspirational music in the background will aid in having the self-hypnotic trance take a deeper effect.

THE PHYSIOTHERAPY TECHNIQUE™ (continued)

Recite The Following Prayer Audibly:

To ward off depression, pain and negativity, I make the sign of the cross and then affirm, " by this sign I conquer." You demons, you devil – let go, because I let God. I call on the power of divine restoration. My good of past and present is divinely restored to me now. This is a time of divine fulfillment. I give thanks for my divine restoration in mind, body, financial affairs, and in all my relationships. I am in God's hands, under God's power, for I am certainly God's property now.

I will also memorize the following prayer, reciting it often: "Count it all joy, my brethren, when you meet various trials, for you know that the testing of your faith produces steadfastness. And let steadfastness have its full effect, that you may be perfect and complete, lacking in nothing." (James 1: 2-4)

If you happened to think the The Physiotherapy Technique has nothing to do with hypnotism, you would be dead wrong. In fact, exercise is one of the most effective ways to acquire the discipline to stay focused, in addition to becoming relaxed, physically and mentally. Think: "Exercise, Exorcism."

The closer a person comes to relaxing under meditation the closer that person is able to reach the unfathomable powers that reside latent within the subconscious. Actually, during mediation, and after exercising, the brain waves become very much the same as when undergoing hypnosis. This means that the person who practices meditating, and has exercised is more prepared to be hypnotized than the one who has not practiced. It may seem strange, but I sometimes suggest exercise for exorcism to my patients.

When committing to The Physiotherapy Technique you will receive a multitude of benefits. First and foremost, is the surprising sense of high esteem; then comes the feeling of having excessive energy; then comes an increase in strength and endurance; and finally comes the state of total relaxation, and security. The real surprise will come when you realize that you cannot do without the exercises. Upon reaching this point, you will have developed an athletic heart, in more ways then one. You may even come to realize that the pleasure derived from exercise can run a close parallel to having sex. Yes, exercise can become that profound, and enjoyable.

(continue)

THE PHYSIOTHERAPY TECHNIQUE™ (continued)

What Eventually Occurs During This Training

Without exercise, the body tends to degenerate before its time – the spine loses its posture, muscles lose elasticity, and the blood tends to lose its hemoglobin count. Then the spirit begins to yield to negative symptoms, such as high anxiety, neurosis – even complete exhaustion. By exercising, these symptoms can become reversed; conditions such as Chronic Fatigue Syndrome (CFS) can become totally mitigated. Even fear, causing headaches, nausea, ulcers, and various other disorders can become reversed. Since fear feeds the muscle tension that causes many disorders, the key is to alleviate the symptoms. This is achieved by going to the heart of the cause, discovering the reason and then resolving, or redefining, the pattern. Soon afterward, the symptoms would, more than likely, subside.

What does The Physiotherapy Technique have to do with this? Everything! Without going into the vast array of issues associated with exercise, insecurity, and other issues, the important thing is to realize that this therapy can provide a profound positive effect on the many challenges in life. Take the issue of security as an example. Once the feeling of physical and mental relaxation is ascertained, the body begins responding in a totally different way. Then, in adjusting to this renewed sense of security, it induces positive, psychosomatic reactions. When everything feels right, it is likely everything will go smoothly. Putting everything said in perspective, the key to positive transformation really boils down to attitude.

Actually, attitude became the contributing factor behind naming this section. For, in combining these exercises with prayer and affirmations and then linking it all to hypnotherapy, it becomes a physiological experience producing harmony, unity, and purpose within the participant. The purpose for this orchestrated approach is so that it will provide conformity, change, and eventually the complete transformation of the participant's behavior, especially where attitude is concerned. After a short period, the subject will begin to experience a shift from being anxious and tense, to a state of mental balance and harmony.

Because of replacing negative behavior with this positive activity the heart will respond, producing a smooth, coherent rhythm. This, in turn, has a positive effect on the neurological, autonomic and hormonal activity.

(continue)

THE PHYSIOTHERAPY TECHNIQUE™ (continued)

What Eventually Occurs During This Training (continued)

Additionally, by providing renewed circulatory activity, the muscles become relaxed due to being revitalized with the increased blood circulation.
Not only does exercise serve as a form of exorcism, as well as providing security, it also acts to give the body muscle tone, strong bones, and flexibility within the joints. When our joints become limber, there becomes a probability of alleviating the symptoms of arthritis; or even curing arteriosclerosis – that debilitating disease leading to the thickening and hardening of arterial walls.

Through exercise, the body reacts and serves to force poison, lymphatic fluids, and waste from the muscle tissues, into the blood and to the excretory glands. In addition, exercise serves to aid in strengthening the will, rejuvenation of the cells, organs, skin, and the entire endocrine system, as well as improving the thought and mental patterns of the brain – the most important organ for sustaining life and **longevity**.

THE PHYSIOTHERAPY TECHNIQUE™ (continued)
PHYSIOTHERAPY ABDOMINAL BREATHING

Note: Before beginning any of the exercises listed below, practice the following breathing exercise to experience just how natural breathing occurs. Afterward, you should always apply this technique as a warm-up exercise prior to working out.

To practice <u>Physiotherapy Abdominal Breathing</u> (diaphragmatic breathing), become seated comfortably and place the left hand on the abdomen and the right hand on the chest. Breathe in and out through the nose several times to get the lungs going. Then, with no movement under the right hand, inhale and exhale deeply. With the left hand rising and falling keep breathing in and out, feeling the abdomen expanding and depleting itself of air. When you feel abdomen pushing and falling under the left hand, think of the diaphragm acting as a bellows pushing the air out, and then drawing it in again.

While breathing in, get the feel of your belly enlarging as you hold your left hand firmly against it. While exhaling, push the air out until the abdomen is completely flat. In doing so, make sure the chest remains still under the right hand. After some practice you will begin breathing correctly, perhaps for the first time. This is the professional technique used to teach singers, as well as speakers, as to how to project their voices. To avoid becoming conscious of breathing while exercising, the main rule is to breathe in before initiating the exercise, and then exhale upon completion. To practice this breathing technique, simply lie down in the prone position and repeatedly inhale and exhale using long, deep breaths.

<u>Physiotherapy Abdominal Breathing</u> will happen automatically within the diaphragm because of the natural function of the Sympathetic Nervous System.

THE PHYSIOTHERAPY TECHNIQUE™ (continued)
PHYSIOTHERAPY IMAGRY

Many people have difficulty perceiving themselves as having a great body. Some people have trouble addressing being overweight, while others are preoccupied by the fact that their physical condition doesn't measure up to their own standards. Still others procrastinate about doing anything at all to improve their self-image. The following self-hypnosis induction has been designed to alter negative attitudes, in addition to instilling new ways of gaining optimism and self-esteem.

Through Physiotherapy Imagery, persons become enabled to imagine the old self in a new light simply by "reframing," (projecting the transformed ideal self, subconsciously). Before proceeding with the prescribed scripts below, follow the self-hypnosis procedure as described previously. It is advisable to practice going into self-hypnosis at least four times a week. Always strive to reach your ideal physical condition keeping a positive image while practicing self-hypnosis during makeover exercise. The inductions shown below are examples of the use of self-hypnosis for positive transformation. Whether it is the subject, the patient, or the hypnotherapist taping hypnotic scripts for improvement, this is an extremely effective way to unleash the power of the subconscious mind.   After taping the following induction, *"Go Into" The Trance Zone*, and listen to the words until satisfactory results are achieved.

IMAGERY MAKEOVER HYPNOSIS SCRIPT - REFRAMING

SUBJECT, Or PATIENT: (sitting, lying, or kneeling)

"Go Into" The Trance Zone, then proceed.

Now, breathing in deeply, I take in full breaths as if I can picture the oxygen filling my lungs. As I continue to breathe deeply, I imagine the oxygen as a magic healing vapor. The deeper I breathe, the deeper this healing vapor circulates into my entire body. The more oxygen I take in, the more I feel the effect of its healing powers. I can visualize a clear picture of this healing vapor going into my lungs and circulating throughout my nervous system. I imagine every part of my body becoming so relaxed it seems like jelly. I allow this magic healing vapor to relieve every pain, every arthritic condition, every restrictive feeling in my body. I allow this magic vapor to balance my entire nervous system, my complete immune system, as I focus on allowing my mind to come to complete rest. I am free of all worry, free of all anxiety and stress as I drift deep into my hypnotic trance.

(continued)

IMAGERY MAKEOVER HYPNOSIS SCRIPT - REFRAMING SUBJECT, Or PATIENT:

Deeper and deeper I go into this deep trance state; deeper and deeper I go into hypnosis. The deeper I go into hypnosis, the deeper I go into this trance state. Deeper and deeper, I drift deeper into my transforming, hypnotic trance. Still using my imagination, I can visualize myself in my present condition inside a large, black frame with all my present features shown in black and white. Suddenly, in my imagination, I see this picture dissolve. Then, I reappear inside of a large, silver screen with my image in vivid color. In a television-like window, I have become larger than life with my complete figure appearing quite colorful. As I visualize myself removing my clothes and standing in my underwear, I study the features of my entire body.

I am pleased with this image, but in order to appear even better, I imagine myself with a desirable body, having a figure I can really feel proud about. As I envision the changes taking place, I can see my muscle tone developing and becoming more appealing to my eyes. Now, I can actually begin see the way I might look after doing some physical exercises. Although I feel some changes taking place right now, I know that I am beginning to look great, feeling better at every moment. This amazing transformation is occurring now, and will happen every time I recall this exercise as I "Go Into" The Trance Zone.

As I keep focused on this very appealing image of myself, I can see that I have developed an attractive body, with my weight finally being to where it should be for my height. As I stare, admiring myself to the point I can actually accept this as this true, I can imagine myself as I appeared in my clothes. Now, as I envision myself in a new set of clothes, I marvel at how appealing I look in these new clothes, and how attractive I have become through this positive transformation. I find this quite intriguing as I allow these images of my renewed self become etched, pleasingly, in my mind.

Using my imagination once again, I study the entire picture of myself inside this silver screen. And as I focus on my image, I see the whole scene becoming even more life-like. As I continue to focus and imagine how great I look, I admire this great image of my newly developed persona. As I focus on this enlarged image, I begin counting from one to three: 1 . . . I replace the bright silver screen with a splendid, gilded frame. 2 . . . And finding myself appearing in an appealing full portrait pose. 3 . . . Since this gilded frame presents my portrait similar to those expensive frames for masterpieces in museums, it becomes engraved in my subconscious mind.   (continued)

<u>IMAGERY MAKEOVER HYPNOSIS SCRIPT - REFRAMING</u>
<u>SUBJECT, Or PATIENT:</u>

Now, this image of myself has found a permanent place in my mind, and I am able to call upon this ideal self-portrait any time I wish. With my newly formed identity, I now envision myself as the person I've always dreamed I could be. In this state of subconscious, I can always recall how great it felt to have my imagination make me over. My subconscious mind has allowed me see and feel this greatly improved image of myself. When I come out of this trance, I will remember everything that has taken place, and will be able to reflect on it every time I wish to improve my image. Whether I reflect on it, or not, this session is already taking a positive affect on me – and it will continue to do so in real time, automatically.

By the time I count from one to five, I will open my eyes feeling alert, refreshed, and alive. 1 . . . 2 . . . Every part of me is positive and feeling confident in every way. 3 . . . I am feeling ten times better about myself. 4 . . . I have become filled with self-esteem. 5 . . . I have overcome being self-conscious about my weight. I am fully alive as I open my eyes.

THE PHYSIOTHERAPY TECHNIQUE™ (continued)
PHYSIOTHERAPY EXERCISES

The exercises, as described below, consist of a combination of effective anaerobic, aerobic and resistance techniques that have taken years of sweat to develop. Any "kinks" have been modified and rectified thereby producing selectively balanced, well organized "sets," or groups of highly effective exercises. One of the best things about this Physiotherapy Technique ™ is that there is no fancy, or expensive, equipment involved. A ten pound dumbbell and a mat is all that is required to perform any, or all, of the exercises - a fantastic benefit for those having little space to work from. No matter whether you are looking for performance, bodybuilding, athletic ability or merely becoming physically fit, the following exercises will, certainly, fulfill your needs. For sure, the more you work at this, the more you will be amazed at the results.

Although these exercises are designed to greatly improve the physical condition, be sure not to neglect other exercises, such as walking, swimming, tennis, bicycling, etc. - the main objective is to find ways of becoming motivated, to strive to become physically and mentally fit, no matter what that takes. No matter which kind of program you select to become fit, be sure to drink at least 6 to 8 glasses of water daily. Not only does this prevent dehydration, but it also washes away the many unwanted toxins, and free radicals that continuously invade the body. It is okay to drink water when exercising, but not advisable to add ice.

An Important Note About Exercise

When most people think about exercise they shirk from the idea of doing them for two reasons: 1 – They think they will become too tired; 2 – They think exercise will take away the energy they need to do other things. In both cases they are gravely (and I use the term loosely), misinformed. The amazing truth about exercise is that it provides more energy – the more you participate, the more the energy builds up. The day you begin to exercise is the day you reverse becoming tired. In the days following, you will find you have such access energy you will become astounded by how many tasks you begin taking on – not to mention the enthusiasm it brings (okay, so I mentioned it). You owe it to yourself to begin exercising your way to progressive health – otherwise it soon becomes digressive. Especially invigorating are the following exercises: Walking, running, swimming, Shadow-boxing, jumping rope and deep knee bends. **See Illustration 14 - 4 below**.

THE PHYSIOTHERAPY TECHNIQUE™ (continued)
THE ILLUSTRATIONS

When performing these exercises, bear in mind two things: First – always strive to increase the repetitions until reaching your comfort zone. Second – although these exercises have a specific order, keep experimenting until you find which exercises give the best results, predicated by your intuitive feelings.

Note: After becoming familiar with the exercises, you may feel more comfortable by alternating the First Set of Exercises one day, and the Second Set of Exercises the next day. Although it may make sense to deviate from the sequences due to the needs the body requires, it is crucial to always begin with the Warm Up Exercises.

Warm Up Exercises - Standing Up
Activates the lungs and stretches the muscles of the upper torso. **14 – 1 Swimstroke** -- continue with closed fingers – **1 minute**. **14 – 2 Alternating Fists** continue with closed fists – **1 minute.**

When doing these Warm Up Exercises spend 1 minute on each of the exercises as illustrated. (Complete these without resting.)

Warm Up Exercises

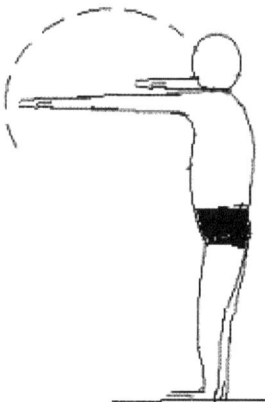

Illustration 14 – 1   Swimstroke

Begin with the Swimstroke by shifting the arms above the head and thrusting forward, imitating the overhand swimming stroke. Keep the fingers together. **Repeat this exercise for 1 minute.**

THE ILLUSTRATIONS
Warm Up Exercises (continued)

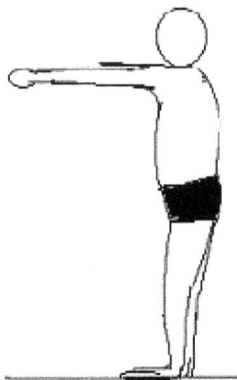

Illustration 14 – 2 Alternating Fists

Continue with the Alternating Fists by bringing the hands to the shoulders and making fists. Then thrust each fist forward, alternating them, as they are thrust forward and back, as if punching an invisible bag. During this exercise think of it as a flowing motion in two stages: 1 - while keeping the chest erect, pivot at the waist and count 5 strokes smiling and exhaling making a hiss sound. 2 - continue with another count of 5 strokes, while inhaling with the mouth puckered making a sucking sound. This type of breathing causes the lungs to become purified, as well as increasing the lung capacity. The smile aids in keeping everything positive, and energized. Doing this also helps to intensify concentration, for any purpose. Keep the fingers closed into a fist.

Repeat this exercise for 1 minute.

THE ILLUSTRATIONS (continued)
First Set of Exercises

First Set of Exercises - Standing Up
14 – 3 Alternate Kick – Begin this set with **10 kicks** each leg. **14 – 4 Deep Knee Bend** – Repeat this exercise **10 times.** **14 – 5 Elephant Swing** – For limbering up - **frequently** **14 – 6 Touch Toes Straight** – Repeat this exercise **10 times.** **14 – 7 Touch Opposite Toes** – Repeat this exercise **10 times.** **14 – 8 Dumbbell Curl & Press** – Repeat this exercise **10 times.**

When doing this First Set of Exercises, as illustrated below, Repeat each one as specified, then gradually increase the repetitions as you progress. Note: As with all these exercises, keep increasing the repetitions until reaching your ideal physical condition. Always take several minutes rest between exercises.

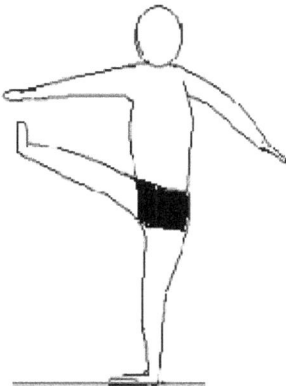

Illustration 14 –3 Alternate Kick

Begin this set of exercises with the feet flat on the floor. Then, balancing on the left foot, extend the left hand straight out, and try to kick the extended left palm with the right foot. Continue by switching legs, balancing on the right foot. Now, extend the right hand straight out, and try to kick the extended right palm with the left foot. Not only is this exercise excellent for stamina, weight control, circulation, and posture, it is an excellent way of gaining profound mental and physical equilibrium.

Repeat this exercise 10 times.

THE ILLUSTRATIONS
First Set of Exercises (continued)

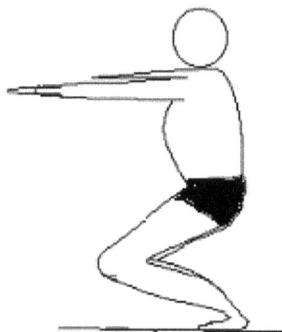

Illustration 14 – 4   Deep Knee Bend

To execute this exercise, begin by standing with the feet shoulder width flat on the floor. Then, with the hands extended palms down, the eyes looking straight ahead, keep the spine straight and let the torso drop as you bend the knees. Done properly, this will place you in the ideal bending position, balancing on your toes. Then, still balancing on your toes, rise up to the original standing position until the feet become flat on the floor again. **Repeat this exercise 10 times.**

Note: Since brain cells die at the rate of millions per second, this form of breathing enables the oxygen to replenish the brain cells at a more intensified rate. When breathing, think of breathing between the eyes while breathing through the nose. Not only does breathing in this manner act to replenish the brain cells, but doing this special deep-knee exercise serves to improve the condition of the blood's capillaries, as well.

When performing this exercise, the immune system becomes inundated with such an abundance of oxygen, the brain, as well as the respiratory and circulatory systems become revitalized. And since capillaries are a vital part of the blood, providing the body with this kind of oxygen replenishment goes a long way toward altering the molecular structure, as well as rejuvenating the immune system. Although this exercise may cause hyperventilation, which could cause dizziness, try to stick with it. Try starting with fewer repetitions, and then increase them, gradually.

THE ILLUSTRATIONS
First Set of Exercises (continued)

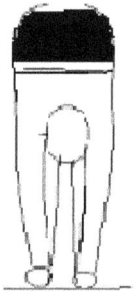

Illustration 14 – 5 Elephant Swing

For limbering up in preparation for the next several exercises bend over, letting the head and hands hang freely. Then, gently bouncing, pivot at the waist and continue bouncing from side to side. This exercise is not only good for relaxation, but the flow of blood becomes invigorating for the head and scalp. Do this for **1 minute**. **Repeat this exercise 2 times.**

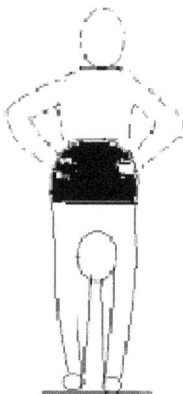

Illustration 14 – 6 Touch Toes Straight

Beginning from a standing position with the hands on the hips, and the feet spread shoulder width, bend straight down and touch the toes. Bending over, and stretching as far as possible each time try to touch the fingers to the toes. With every repetition, strive to stretch far enough to have bent fists touch the floor between the feet. For most people, this will take many attempts. However, never force when stretching. The object is to practice until the muscles become loose enough so that they stretch more and more over time. This exercise is especially good for stamina, weight control and circulation. It fact, this serves to greatly improve the posture. **Repeat this exercise 10 times.**

THE ILLUSTRATIONS
First Set of Exercises (continued)

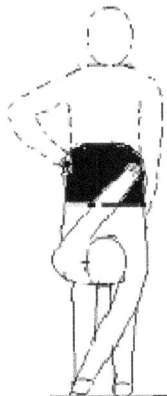

Illustration 14 – 7 Touch OppositeToes

Beginning from a standing position with the hands on the hips, and the feet spread shoulder width, bend down and stretch either hand to touch the opposite toes. When bending over each time, alternate the hands and stretch as far as possible trying to touch the fingers to the opposite toes. Pivot at the waist to get as much motion as possible. This exercise is especially good for the abdomen and vital organs, as well as the chest and arm muscles. This also serves to greatly improve the posture. **Repeat this exercise 10 times.**

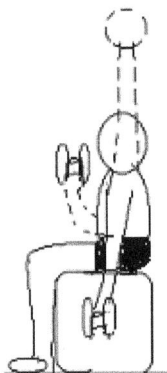

Illustration 14– 8 Dumbbell Curl / Press

Using only <u>one ten-pound dumbbell</u>, become seated and lift it (in either hand) to shoulder height, then straight above the head. Performed in two sweeping motions, lift the dumbbell up to the shoulder, then twist the wrist forward and lift it straight above the head. When dropping down to the shoulder twist the wrist again and drop the hand to the side. This action serves to strengthen the combined muscles of the arms, hands, wrists, and shoulders. **Repeat this exercise 7 times.**

THE ILLUSTRATIONS
Second Set of Exercises

Take a **Brief Rest** before proceeding to the **Second Set of Exercises.**
Always take several minutes to rest between exercises.

Note: Keep experimenting, eliminating some exercises one day and doubling up on others the next. Keep striving to reach your ideal physical condition.

Second Set of Exercises - Practiced On Floor
14 – 9 Rowing and Alternate – Repeat this combined exercise **2 times.**
14 – 10– Alternate Leg Swings – Repeat this exercise **10 times.**
14 – 11 Half Sit Ups – Repeat this exercise **10 times.**

In doing this **Second Set of Exercises**, as illustrated below, **Repeat** each one as specified then gradually increase the repetitions as you progress.

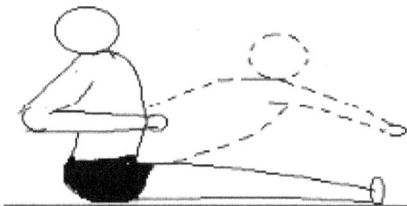

Illustration 14 – 9 Rowing & Alternate

Beginning in a sitting position, stretch both hands forward, reach to touch the toes with the fingertips, and continuing in a flowing motion, pull the arms backwards while making fists until the back becomes arched. Do this as if rowing a boat.
Do this exercise **5 times**.

Next, placing the left hand behind the back, stretch the right hand over to the left foot and reach to touch the left toe with the fingertips, and continuing in a sweeping motion, pull the arm back making a fist, and place it behind the back. Then continue the same procedure using the left hand.
Do this **5 times**. This combination is especially good for breathing and stamina.

Repeat this combined exercise 2 times.

THE ILLUSTRATIONS
Second Set of Exercises (continued)

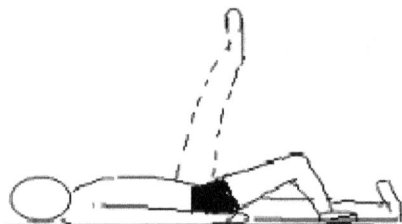

Illustration 14 – 10 Alternate Leg Swing

While lying in a comfortable position with the hands resting at the sides bend the right leg and lock the knee and foot into position. Then, swing the left leg as high as possible while keeping the leg straight, extending the toes forward. Upon bringing the leg down keeping it straight and bending the toes back toward the knee, let the leg drop, stopping it just before the foot touches the floor. Continue the exercise by switching to the opposite leg. When swinging each leg, scissors-like, concentrate on the pivotal action of the hip, ankle and foot muscles.
Repeat this exercise 10 times.

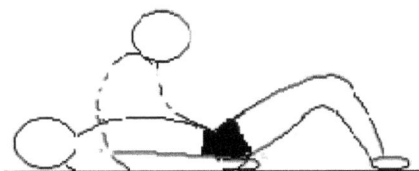

Illustration 14 – 11 Half Sit Ups

Lying in a comfortable position with the hands resting at the sides, raise the chest, keeping the neck straight. When doing this Half Sit Ups exercise, keep the hands flat, and the knees bent and locked into position. In addition to strengthening the spine, this exercise is great for tightening the abdominal muscles.
Repeat this exercise 10 times.

THE PHYSIOTHERAPY TECHNIQUE™ (continued)
THE ILLUSTRATIONS

The Human Blossom – Cleansing Exercise (Optional)
14 – 12A Inhale – Begin with **Inhale** in the fetus position. **14 – 12B Exhale** – After rising up **Exhale** while returning to the fetus position.

THE HUMAN BLOSSOM – CLEANSING EXERCISE:
The Human Blossom is performed as a two-fold exercise as demonstrated:

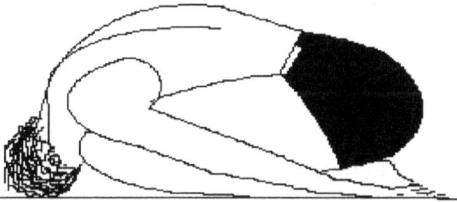

Illustration 14 – 12A Inhale:

In the fetus position as shown above in **Illustration 14 – 12A**, take in several breaths to relax. Then, **Inhale** while reciting the following affirmation:
Out with demons; out with disease; out with all debilitating negativity.

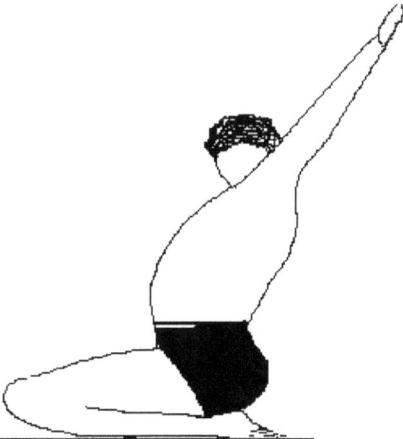

Illustration 14 – 12B Exhale:
After reaching the chest-expansion position with the hands above the head as shown above in **Illustration 14 – 12B**, begin to **Exhale** while lowering the arms and reciting the following prayer:
In with God's Supernatural Power; In with the spirit of Jesus Christ.
Perform this exercise 5 times a week.

THE HUMAN BLOSSOM – CLEANSING TRANCE

For added protection against all evil forces, recite the following prayer audibly at least once a week in the **The Human Blossom** position. (Optional)

Either practice memorizing *The Whole Armor of God,* or read it the following page aloud as you *"Go Into"* *The Trance Zone*. Yes, oddly enough, going into the trance zone can be done while reading with the eyes open.

SUBJECT, Or PATIENT

I am fortunate because I am in harmony with the universe of abundance, which is in perfect sync with the powers of my creator and His Divine plans for me. I shall reinforce this fact by reciting:

Finally, my brethren, be strong in the Lord, and in the power of His Might. Put on the whole armor of God that you may be able to stand against the wiles of the devil. For we wrestle not with flesh and blood, but against principalities, against powers, against rulers of darkness of this world, against spiritual wickedness in high places.

Wherefore take unto you the whole armor of God that you may be able to withstand in the evil day, and having done all, to stand. Stand, therefore, having your loins girt about with truth, and having on the breastplate of righteousness; and having your feet shod with the preparation of the gospel of peace.

Above all, taking the shield of faith wherewith you shall be able to quench all the fiery darts of the wicked.

And take the helmet of salvation, and the sword of the Spirit, which is the word of God, praying always in the Spirit, and watching for all saints.

. . . Ephesians 6: 10 - 18

PHYSIOTHERAPY TECHNIQUE ™

REVIEW:

Through a never-ending responsibility to ourselves, we must see to it that our bodies get the proper exercise and nourishment, enough so that it becomes a sustaining fuel – a progressive blood / cell regeneration process. This physical conditioning is our only way of retarding the inevitable pull towards death.

In fact, in the animal kingdom the expression "survival of the fittest" is truly representative of their way of life. In their world, the weak are always the first to succumb. Ironically, it is the same in our world: "inevitable death" holds a ringside seat and continues to beckon the underdog called "self-neglect," while lasting life, the opponent as "the fittest," spars to claim the title of <u>longevity</u>. The exercises listed above are not only intended to improve the quality of life for those willing to participate, but they also insure that total fitness includes a sound mind, healthy body and a positive spirit so as to serve as that corridor to long life

<u>Exercise / Exorcism</u>: For many persons, exercise is a dirty word, an activity to be avoided at all costs. Of those few, I can only add that exercise can act as a form of exorcism, so be careful of what you <u>don't wish for,</u> as this kind of avoidance could become dangerous to your health. Remember: Exorcise is Exorcism. Be smart: Choose Exercise as the right path to spiritual health – choose aerobic or anaerobic exercise <u>you can live with</u> – literally.

REVIEW:

By providing renewed circulatory activity, the muscles become relaxed due to being revitalized with the increased blood circulation. Not only does exercise serve as a form of exorcism, as well as providing security, it also acts to give the body muscle tone, strong bones, and flexibility within the joints. When our joints become limber, there becomes a probability of alleviating the symptoms of arthritis; or even curing arteriosclerosis – that debilitating disease leading to the thickening and hardening of arterial walls.

Through exercise, the body reacts and serves to force poison, lymphatic fluids, and waste from the muscle tissues, into the blood and to the excretory glands. In addition, exercise serves to aid in strengthening the will, rejuvenation of the cells, organs, skin, and the entire endocrine system, as well as improving the thought and mental patterns of the brain – the most important organ for sustaining life and <u>longevity</u>.

. . . EJL

TO END ON A POSITIVE NOTE
Ponder These Final Thoughts:

To Love Is To Radiate

Love *is a spirit: As an electrical energy it is the unseen chemical element, which transcends like a current as it carries each molecule to its destination. In the body this chemical process is also known as "body fluids" – in the universe it is called "interplanetary expansion." The only way to control your moods and feelings is through your thoughts. What you think is what you are, and eventually what you will become. What you fill your mind with is what will influence you in your relationships and throughout your life.*

Love *is that positive force which, when applied, is capable of creating the impossible, but when opposed and completely reversed to the negative force, hate, it is capable of much havoc and destruction. Radiate pure love, and you will illuminate the people around you, attracting them like an irresistible magnet.*

YES – Your Everlasting Spirit

People are forever telling you, NO. It may come from Your friend, Your neighbor, Your enemy, Your boss, Your associate, Your spouse, Your child, or even Your brother. Well, now it's time to think Y.E.S.!

Human nature, itself, warrants prejudice against the positive: It will try to win out because of the pull of the negative, opposing pole. There is also the pull between good and evil, ups and downs, male and female, success and failure – That's just life. But, who said life was Just.

The only way to combat these opposing forces is to gain faith. Faith will give you the foundation, The Seed, The Will, The Confidence, and The Desire to have everything Go Your Way. There is no mystery here – Opposition always requires defense, and defense must be achieved by Complete Preparation.

That Preparation is Faith: A belief in The Power Stronger than the self. And That Power is beyond life – It Is The Power of The Holy Spirit.

. . . EJL

CHAPTER FOURTEEN
14

THE TRANCE ZONE
HYPNOTHERAPY COURSE

---

14 HYPNOTHERAPY COURSE
CERTIFICATION:

*After working as a hypnotherapist for over fifteen years and treating patients
based on his book, "The Trance Zone Hypnosis Manual,"
Edward J Longo realized he had developed enough material for a 2nd book.
This became:
The Trance Zone Hypnotherapy Course, Hypnotherapy Certification –
The Book For Hypnotists, Hypnotherapists, and Practitioners.*

                                        . . . EJL

CHAPTER FOURTEEN

14

THE TRANCE ZONE HYPNOTHERAPY
COURSE & CERTIFICATION

THE FUTURE OF HYPNOTHERAPY

Alternative Therapy Of The Future:

Physicians prescribing medicine or doctors targeting treatment to specific regions of the brain will not make hypnotherapy become obsolete. Quite the contrary, it is only a matter of time before The Trance Zone Hypnotherapy will change the psychological, physiological and spiritual aspects of patients for the better. In fact, research has already proven that cognitive therapy, without drugs, improves the brain function of persons who were diagnosed with OCD. Given that cognitive therapy serves to transform the brain, then because hypnosis is so effective at bringing subconscious behaviors to the fore hypnotherapy would be a very potent form of cognitive therapy. Although hypnosis had previously received a bad reputation, it has become so widely accepted that it is now unlikely it will ever regress into such terrible disrepute. Compared to rising medical costs, surgery and hospital stays, hypnotherapy remains inexpensive while its results are amazingly effective, and long lasting.

After working as a hypnotherapist and treating patients for upwards of fifteen years based on his book, "*The Trance Zone Hypnosis Manual*," the author realized he had developed enough material for his 3rd book. This newly released book became:

Integrative Medicine The Professional Guide to Mental Health and Positive Transformation.

THE TRANCE ZONE HYPNOTHERAPY COURSE

After taking the initial step of ordering The Trance Zone Hypnosis Manual the candidate can seriously consider becoming a Certified Hypnotherapist. Due to all the damaging, negative influences bombarding us from all fronts Hypnotherapists within this health related field are becoming quite respected, and more in demand.

In addition to valuable information leading to legitimate Hypnotherapy certification, Edward J Longo, an approved hypnotherapy college instructor, provides private sessions of hands-on instruction. Each candidate will be informed of professional services, which include physical, spiritual and mental therapy. Expert advice, including remedies will be introduced for anxiety disorders, panic attacks, depression, mental abuse, bipolar, mania, personality disorders, physical and mental dysfunction, OCD, phobias, memory loss, stress, and other health issues. All Major Mental Disorders as per the Surgeon General's Health Report will be introduced, reviewed and addressed during the private sessions. Indeed, due to the extensive background of this master hypnotherapy instructor, much insight will be provided.

Fortunately, there is a hypnotherapy course that provides vital information on alleviating many mental disorders. This hypnotherapy course is appropriately named: The Trance Zone Hypnotherapy Course.

The Trance Zone Hypnosis Manual *for* Hypnotherapy Certification
www.thetrancezone.com

The good news is that this course can be completed in less than five short months. A handsome, legitimate Hypnotherapy Certificate suitable for framing will be provided upon completing the Tests Examinations.

For More Information Review the
INQUIRY FORM below

THE TRANCE ZONE
HYPNOTHERAPY COURSE
E-MAIL INQUIRY FORM

Yes! I want to benefit from your Hypnotherapy Course, which I understand may be approved by the American Board of Hypnotherapy. I also understand that after I receive your certification I will automatically be able to qualify for the prestigious certificate offered by American Board of Hypnotherapy.

Please print my name on your Certificate as follows:
_____

Please check the appropriate choices below:

(_) I am interested in enrolling after January, 2013, which will include your certification. I also understand I will receive *The Trance Zone Hypnosis Manual* upon enrollment.
(_) Please provide information regarding your certification course listed below.
The Trance Zone Hypnotherapy Course - Hypnotherapy Certification, and Hypnosis and Hypnotherapy, A Psychotherapist's Guide To Positive Transformation.

Note that the complete certification course may also be taken Online, by mail, or by Email. Certification will be provided after satisfactory completion of the Hypnotherapy Course.

Name & Title: _____

Address: _____ City:_____ State_____

Country: USA – or Other: _____-____

Phone: _____ Email: _____

Brief Background: _____ Date: _____

===

PLEASE PRINT and submit by snail mail, or
COPY & PASTE and e-mail the above form to:
Affinity@affinityzone.com

HOW TO BECOME A GIFTED CERTIFIED HYPNOTHERAPTIST

The Six Keys:

1. Practice, then experiment, and then implement all the knowledge and insight gained . . . .

2. Apply all therapy treatments in a compassionate, caring, and honest manner . . . .

3. Establish a bond while relaxing the subject with smooth, soothing, positive WORDS . . .

4. Gain trust by presenting positive suggestions, and by gaining subject's trust. . . . . .

5. Guide, lead, and direct the subject through guided imagery through truth and positive focus . . . . .

6. Create an Atmosphere of trust using the 3 S's: Soundness, Sincerity, and Smoothness of voice.

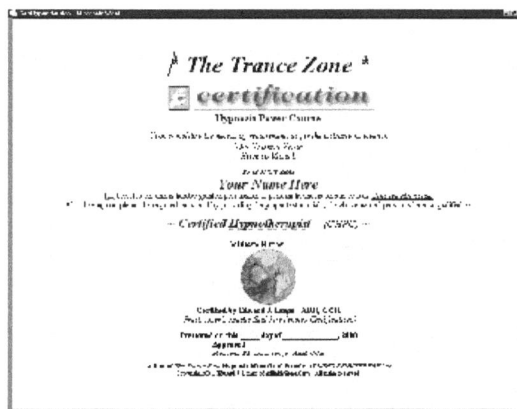

SAMPLE CERTIFICATE

Continue below for further information on becoming a legitimate, board certified professional hypnotherapist

CONTACT INFORMATION

Credentialed Certification with the following Organizations:
American Board of Hypnotherapy (ABH)
American College of Hypnotherapy (ACH)
American Association of Behavioral Therapists (RBT)
American Association of Psychotherapists. (AAP)

The Trance Zone Hypnotherapy Course
To find out how to qualify to become a Certified Hypnotherapist,
Or to review other products, visit the website links below.
Send E-Mails To: master@affinityzone.com

Featured Hypnotherapy Link
http://www.thetrancezone.com

Edward J Longo - ABH CCH RBT
503 East 78th Street, New York, NY 10075 (212) 737-8538
Founder: Affinity Zone www.affinityzone.com
Founder: The Trance Zone Hypnotherapy School
Author / Instructor: The Trance Zone Hypnosis Manual
Website URL: http://www.thetrancezone.com

Think CAREER!

Become a Certified Hypnotherapist using The Trance Zone Hypnosis Manual.

The Trance Zone Hypnosis Manual is really priceless because persons can actually become professional hypnotherapists merely by implementing its concepts. As a profession, this is a most rewarding line of work. Even college graduates who wind up spending over $60,000 are not able reach the status, the level of compatibility this hypnosis manual provides. This profession is both extremely challenging, and rewarding because of the gratification that goes with empowering patients, the freedom of being independent, and the respect one receives, socially.

When you purchase *The Trance Zone Hypnosis Manual* you not only learn about self-hypnosis, and how to become an expert at hypnosis, you also begin to apply the course as the entire hypnotherapy foundation - the technique is really that profound. You see, WORDS as positive suggestions are the life-blood of communication, as well as the sparks of transformation. They portray thoughts, feelings, emotions, ideas and ever so much more. They bridge the gap between the conscious and the subconscious, and always provide infinite possibilities. Yet this magical, readily available Secret Weapon is frequently underestimated, and way too often misunderstood. Normally, people love to be engulfed, surrounded, and entertained by words used in stories, speaking, and tales expressed in books. That's why advertising and the media are such booming industries. That's why people read newspapers - it's why people love reading about stories they've experienced themselves. The more the individual can become a confident story teller the more persons will become attracted to that voice, that personality, that entertainer and, in this case, that therapist.

Finally, a respectable way to make more than $1,000 a week in the privacy of your own home! Yes, for many it may be the perfect career! By following his incredible technique as outlined in *The Trance Zone Hypnotherapy Course*, the author, Edward J. Longo, ABH board certified hypnotherapist, will provide information to spark, and possibly launch a gratifying career. As a certified hypnotherapist you will gain recognition in categories such as mental health services, alternative medicine, mind-body medicine, as well as hypnotherapy. By learning how to develop this specialized career the student becomes independent, essentially empowered by such rewarding involvement. And, all this can even be done from the comfort of one's own home. This is a completely documented method of creating a Professional Career, complete with a legitimate certificate.

Think CAREER! (continued)

The Good News is that anyone over the age of 18, regardless of race, gender, or financial standing can become certified to become a practicing hypnotist, or hypnotherapist. More good news is that you don't need to be a college graduate. All the education you need to qualify is based on your own personal life experiences.

In reality, this program is geared to suit each individual, regardless of personal background. Within the next few months you could be on your way to earning more than $50,000 income per year. As amazing as it may seem, hypnotherapist Edward J. Longo will introduce you to a way of achieving all this! Here is your opportunity to apply your insight, your talents, and your beliefs in order to help people. Within three to six months this remarkable course will give you all the tools and expertise required to begin a practice as a Certified Hypnotist, or Hypnotherapist.

❖   **Just think: Getting paid the same day as providing your service! How many careers allow anyone to accomplish this?**

You will find it astonishing to learn that the price for becoming a legally certified hypnotherapist will be less than the cost of just one month's tuition toward any college degree. And the good news is that this course can be completed in less that six short months. Certification will be provided for $225 for two years, $100 per year thereafter. A handsome Hypnotherapy Certificate suitable for framing will be provided upon completing the Examinations. Membership to the American Association of Behavioral Therapists may be free of charge for the first year - another benefit besides the $200 value stated above.

*For many applicants **The Trance Zone Hypnotherapy Course** will be extremely easy because it requires not much experience beyond life experience. Even more good news is that no other experience, courses, credentials, schooling, or degrees are required to begin this course. There are potentially thousands of people in surrounding areas, and elsewhere, where they are suffering from some kind of disorder, or health issue. In essence, because of the worldly problems causing havoc and confusion, the entire world becomes your marketplace. And equally important, this program is not a scam. This program is 100% legal, and a perfect way to professionally make an excellent income year after year. With NO Bosses!*

(continue)

Think CAREER! (continued)

Not only is information provided as to how treat prospective clients there will be many opportunities to experience the rewards and benefits of treating, and transforming them. Soon, there will be immense gratification as more and more clients become established, as well as experiencing the very handsome fee during the process. Sometimes, their only requirement is that they need to listen to a voice delivering positive suggestions.

The Founder EDWARD J. LONGO will demonstrate, step by step, exactly how to become certified as a hypnotherapist. Upon completion of the program in its entirety you will be awarded the legitimate, prestigious Hypnotherapy Certification. The Certificate provided by this Board Certified Hypnotherapist will enable you to treat people, whether they desire to become sound-minded, prosperous, physically healthy, or whether they simply wish to learn how relieve stress. Isn't it about time you developed a rewarding, SPECIALIZED CAREER for yourself? ***Of course, It Is.***

**(For Information regarding The Trance Zone Manual Review
Appendix A, and Appendix B below)**

Appendix A – Hypnotherapy Certification

Phase One Includes the history of hypnosis, self-hypnosis and conditioning, understanding the subconscious mind, how to reach and arouse the Genie within, the Secret 7 Golden Rules, Insight of Mental Energy, structuring successful suggestions, and the ethics of practice. Phase One also includes numerous induction techniques, testing for depth of hypnotic trance, stress tests, and how to treat smoking addiction, obesity, lack of confidence, self-esteem, nail biting, stammering, Tourette's Syndrome, and so much more. Basically, all the technical knowledge one needs to know in order to qualify as a hypnotist is provided using The Trance Zone, one of the most effective hypnosis manuals available anywhere. One reason: being due to its handy pull-out scripts for inducing <u>Hypnotic Trance Scripts</u> to patients.

- **A Brief History of Hypnosis**
- **Functioning As A Hypnotist**
- *The Trance Zone* - **The Concept Behind The Course**
- *The Trance Zone* - **Reaching The Initial State Of Hypnosis**
- **Unleashing The Power Of Your Subconscious Mind**
- **Hypnosis Induction Techniques**

Phase Two Consists of the learned experiences of the certified hypnotist as described above plus the understanding and application of the deep hypnotic states of mind. Here, you will become enabled to address anxiety, health and well being, deepening trance techniques, advanced treatment for specific emotional problems and illnesses, developing and delivering hypnotic scripts, stress management, Spiritual Steam, Electromagnetism, responsibilities of the professional hypnotherapist, (including operating your practice, fees, referrals, etc.,) implanting positive suggestions, including guided imagery enabling you to become a master practitioner. Yes, even becoming empowered physically as well as spiritually, in order to provide health solutions all throughout your career. And finally: registration with the American Board of Hypnotherapy using The Trance Zone Hypnotherapy Certificate as a viable, highly credible credential.

- **Hypnosis Induction Illustrations, Hypnosis Induction**
- **Hypnotist's Posthypnotic Suggestions Induced To Subject**
- **Manifestations of The Highest Kind**
- **Self-Hypnosis Induction Techniques**
- **Self-Hypnosis Induction Illustrations & Self-Hypnosis Behavior**
- **Inducing Majestic Trance Spells**
- **Physiotherapy Technique**

Appendix B

Contents of *The Trance Zone* Hypnosis Manual
(Requirement for Hypnotherapy Certification)

Chapters 1 and 2: Within these pages you will be provided with HISTORICAL FACTS, UNDERSTANDING HYPNOSIS, and EVERYTHING WE ARE COMES FROM THE SUBCONSCIOUS, including some impressive demonstrations. Through the hypnotist, WORDS will paint images on your mind. These images will aid you in mastering control over your life in an ideal, creative way. This chapter reveals the power of hypnosis, as well as the power of imagery. Here you will learn to understand FUNCTION, THE POWER OF HYPNOSIS, THE INSIGHT OF MENTAL IMAGERY, THE CONCEPTION OF MENTAL THOUGHT, and THE SUBJECTS' PERCEPTIBILITY, as well as being provided with a full understanding of hypnosis, and self-hypnosis.

Chapters 3 and 4: In these chapters you will learn, in detail, all the tools necessary for entering the subconscious state of The Trance Zone, including the use of "The Hypnotic Eye." You will also learn about THE PSYSIOLOGY OF *THE TRANCE ZONE*, and THE PSYCHOLOGICAL TOOLS. This chapter provides full induction illustrations on hypnosis and self-hypnosis, including REACHING THE TRANCE ZONE, and THE TRANCE ZONE INDUCTION with many examples of trance scripts and the application thereof.

Chapters 5 and 6: Within these pages you will learn how the mind can alter the brain. They include techniques that will aid in activating the endocrine glands that cause the body to become relaxed, receptive and supple. In this chapter you will learn REPROGRAMMING THE SUBCONSCIOUS MIND, THE MIND CAN ACTUALLY CHANGE THE BRAIN, PHYCHOLOGICAL ADJUSTMENT, PHYSIOLOGICAL ADJUSTMENT, UNLEASHING THE POWER OF THE SUBCONSCIOUS, THE SUBCONSCIOUS GENIE WITHIN, and THE HYPNOSIS. It Boils Down To This: Once you understand and incorporate the power of the subconscious mind, even your most desirable dreams will manifest, as if by magic. These chapters also go into detail explaining the Techniques used to "Go Into" The Trance Zone. In this chapter you will learn many of THE TRANCE ZONE INDUCTION TECHNIQUES, including the application of various kinds of hypnosis trance scripts.

Chapters 7 and 8: These chapters go into detail in explaining the Illustrations used to "Go Into" The Trance Zone. Here you will learn to apply the DEEPER STATE OF TRANCE, such as The Blue Aura Of Dharma Illustration, the Oxygen As An Elixir Illustration, and Behavior Modification Illustration. Also included are demonstrates, in full depth, how the hypnotist successfully hypnotizes the subject through the use of suggestions, and Guided Imagery. In this chapter you will learn about the HYPNOTIST'S INDUCTIONS, and CESSATION OF BAD HABITS (Or Addictions). You will also learn to use important applications such as How To Instill Direction and Motivation.

Contents of *The Trance Zone* Hypnosis Manual (continued)

Chapters 9 and 10: Through examples like learning the Secrets Of Attracting Luck, you will finally come to understand hidden meanings. These are some of the valuable insights introduced in this chapter: TRANCE MANIFESTATIONS, TRANCE-FORMATION VISUALIZER, 7 SECRETS OF ATTRACTING LUCK, and LUCK - The Formula. Here, through the use of the Trance-formation Visualizer, you will learn how to use luck to acquire manifestations of the highest kind. These chapters also demonstrate how the subject successfully induces the complete self-hypnotic Techniques used to "Go Into" The Trance Zone. These inductions have been translated into "the first person" for the convenience of those wishing to use self-hypnosis effectively. In this chapter you will learn to incorporate strategic exercises such as THE TRANCE ZONE INDUCTION TECHNIQUES, and Penetrating The Subconscious Mind

Chapter 11 and 12: These two chapters demonstrate how the subject successfully induces the complete self-hypnotic Illustrations used to "Go Into" The Trance Zone. In this chapter you will learn to apply THE TRANCE ZONE INDUCTION ILLUSTRATIONS, and A DEEPER STATE OF TRANCE such as Behavior Modification Illustration. These inductions have been translated into "the first person" to enable practicing self-hypnosis effectively. Also explained is the special positioning the hands forming "The Observing Eye," and how to induce the highly effective, self-hypnotic, Majestic Trance Spells. Some topics include MAJESTIC TRANCE SPELLS, SUBJECT'S SELF-HYPNOTIC SUGGESTIONS, THE SEVEN DAY TRANCE SPELLS, and DREAM FULFILLMENT DURING SLEEP.

Chapter 13 and 14: Through a special reprogramming process these chapter illustrate, in full detail, specialized mind-altering inductions. For persons desiring to make permanent changes through self-hypnosis, these special inductions will prove highly beneficial. Here are some categories: BEHAVIOR MODIFICATION, REPROGRAMMING THE SUBCONSCIOUS MIND, MIND-ALTERING SUGGESTIONS, and MIND-ALTERING AFFIRMATIONS. Those committing to this UPTT technique will find this as the elixir to the mind and the spirit, as well as the physical body. In doing so, they will be surprised to find it strengthens the will, activates the organs and inspires the spirit. Since exercise is definitely the staple of life, don't hesitate to become fully engaged in The Trance Zone technique. The benefits of this technique will not only prove to be rewarding; they will rekindle your natural desire to live a healthy life. In this final chapter you will learn the value and benefits of A HEALTHY BODY, A SOUND MIND, PHYSIOTHERAPY TECHNIQUE, PHYSIOTHERAPY ABDOMINAL BREATHING, PHYSIOTHERAPY IMAGRY, and PHYSIOTHERAPY EXERCISES and valuable ILLUSTRATIONS.

Note:

The Trance Zone Hypnotherapy Course is certified by
The American Board of Hypnotherapy, and
The American College of Hypnotherapy.

Edward J Longo - Board Certified Clinical Hypnotherapist: *By utilizing the instructions and practicing the applications within* **The Trance Zone Hypnosis Manual***, one can gain access to one's inner programming. The secret to tapping the depths of the mind is to go into the subconscious, where the true source of power rules.   This is where you can unleash the power of the subconscious, and change negative habits of thought and action into what you desire them to be - this is where you can alter your programming for the better.*

When clients learn to incorporate the power of the subconscious mind even their elusive, desirable dreams seem to manifest as if By MAGIC. Through the process of guided imagery, positive suggestions, and deep hypnotic trances, even the most skeptical subjects become influenced.

Testimonial: *Edward J Longo's concept is outstanding, and I recommend The Trance Zone Hypnotherapy Course to anyone who wants to learn to heal themselves, change negative behavioral patterns, or even start a rewarding career as a certified hypnotherapist. I cannot thank Mr. Longo enough for his personal support and mentoring while using his manual throughout my studies. His manual called "The Trance Zone" is the foundation to The Trance Zone Hypnotherapy Course .* **. . . Robin E. Jones – TTZ**

<u>Highly Recommended Reading For Serious Professionals</u>

TRANCE & Treatment *by Herbert Spiegal*
Jung To Live By *by Eugene Pascal, Ph.L*
Imagery In Healing *by Achterberg*
The Neuroscience of Psychotherapy *by Cozolino*
Talk I Not Enough *by Willard Gaylin, M.D*
Your Mental Health *by Allen Frances, M.D*
Your Inner Physician and You *by Upledger*
The Trance Workbook *by Hoffman*
Inner Wisdom & Heal Your Body *by Louise L Hay*
Trance Spells *by Janina Renee*
Tapping The Healer Within *by Callahan*
Acupressure Way of Health *by Teeguarden*
Acupressure Potent Points *by Gach*
Aikido and The Harmony Of Nature *by Saotome*
Clinical Neuropsychology *by Snyder*
DSM-IV Manual of Mental Disorders *4ᵗʰ Edition*
Healing Anxiety & Depression *by Daniel G. Amen, M.D.*
The Trance Zone Hypnosis Manual *by Edward J Longo*
(Edward J Longo – Certified Clinical Hypnotherapy Expert.)

ISBN 978-1-62407-256-7

9 781624 072567

www.ingramcontent.com/pod-product-compliance
Lightning Source LLC
Chambersburg PA
CBHW061415210326
41598CB00035B/6227